BEAT

YOUR

BLOAT

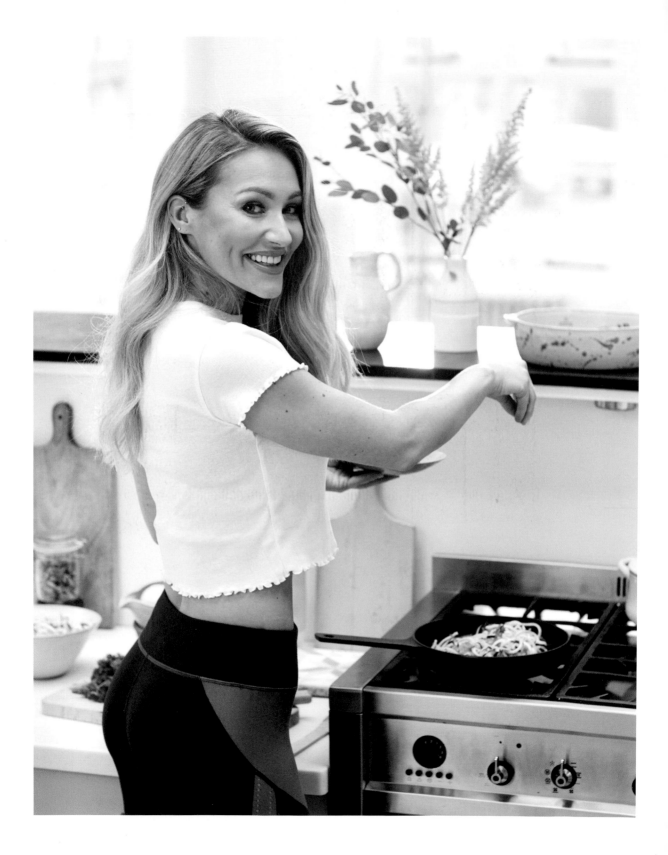

Maeve Madden

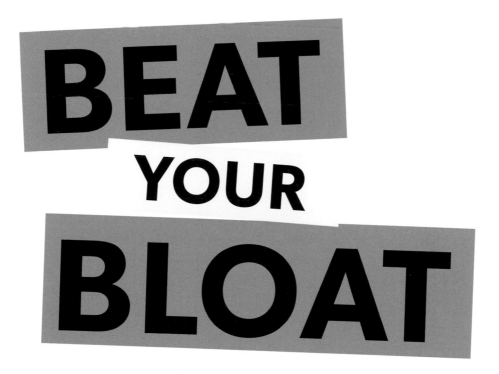

BEAT YOUR BLOAT

Recipes & exercises to promote digestive health

PHOTOGRAPHY BY **CLAIRE PEPPER** AND **TAMIN JONES**

KYLE BOOKS

An Hachette UK Company
www.hachette.co.uk

First published in Great Britain in 2018 by
Kyle Books, an imprint of Kyle Cathie Ltd
Carmelite House
50 Victoria Embankment
London EC4Y 0DZ
www.kylebooks.co.uk

ISBN: 978 0 85783 489 8

Distributed in the US by Hachette Book Group, 1290 Avenue of the Americas,
4th and 5th Floors, New York, NY 10104

Distributed in Canada by Canadian Manda Group, 664 Annette St., Toronto, Ontario, Canada M6S 2C8

Design: Studio nic&lou
Photography: Claire Pepper and Tamin Jones
Food styling: Lizzie Harris
Props styling: Linda Berlin
Production: Lisa Pinnell

A Cataloguing in Publication record for this title is available from the British Library

Printed and bound in Italy

10 9 8 7 6 5 4 3 2 1

Note: The information and advice contained in this book are intended as a general guide.
Neither the author nor the publishers can be held responsible for claims arising from
the inappropriate use of any remedy or exercise regime.
Do not attempt self-diagnosis or self-treatment for serious or long-term conditions before
consulting a medical professional or qualified practitioner. Do not begin any exercise programme
or undertake any self-treatment while taking other prescribed drugs or receiving therapy without
first seeking professional guidance. Always seek medical advice if any symptoms persist.

contents

my story

Hi everyone, I'm Maeve! I am so excited to be able to share with you what I have learnt over the past few years, during which time I've built a positive relationship with myself, with food and my body. I really hope this book helps you to realise that health and fitness are not just about being, and having, the perfect body and lifestyle. No one is perfect and we don't have to try to pretend to be, but we all want to feel confident, strong, happy and beautiful in our own skin. The aim of your lifestyle should simply be to be the best version of yourself.

In 2015, I started sharing my daily life on social media – @maeve_madden – uploading 15-second–1-minute home and gym workout routines. I also posted my favourite delicious recipes, my body transformation from skinny to strong, and tips on how to deal with health conditions like polycystic ovary syndrome (PCOS), irritable bowel syndrome (IBS), small intestinal bacterial overgrowth (SIBO) and adult acne.

I was first diagnosed with PCOS in 2006. I was in my final year at university, writing my dissertation and going through a horrific break-up, and I was definitely not living any kind of healthy lifestyle. I actually don't think I even had gym membership! I had always suffered from irregular periods and when I did go through a menstrual cycle it would be ten days of agonising pain. It felt like there was a world war happening in my uterus – I would be completely drained of energy and I was an emotional, crazy, menstrual mess. Sound familiar? I know I'm not alone! I knew there was something more to this hormonal chaos. Then, while I was writing my dissertation, I collapsed and was rushed to A&E, where I underwent an operation to remove ruptured cysts.

Honestly, I have never quite been the same since. I am not alone in having PCOS; actually, one in 10 women have it – a lot

of them just don't know it. There are so many symptoms of PCOS, which vary from person to person, and they can be really hard to deal with because they can feel embarrassing and make you feel less feminine. My adult acne soon followed, along with problems with weight, bloating, fibroid growth and lack of energy – all because of the hormonal imbalances in my body. Leading a healthy lifestyle, keeping active and eating the right things were – and are – key to my ongoing treatment, and I get ultrasound scans regularly to make sure any potential cysts in my uterus are found and monitored.

For a really long time, I was so angry at my body and couldn't figure out what was wrong and why I was suffering. It wasn't until I posted a picture showing how my body went from lean, toned abs that I worked pretty damn hard for to looking nine months pregnant in a matter of

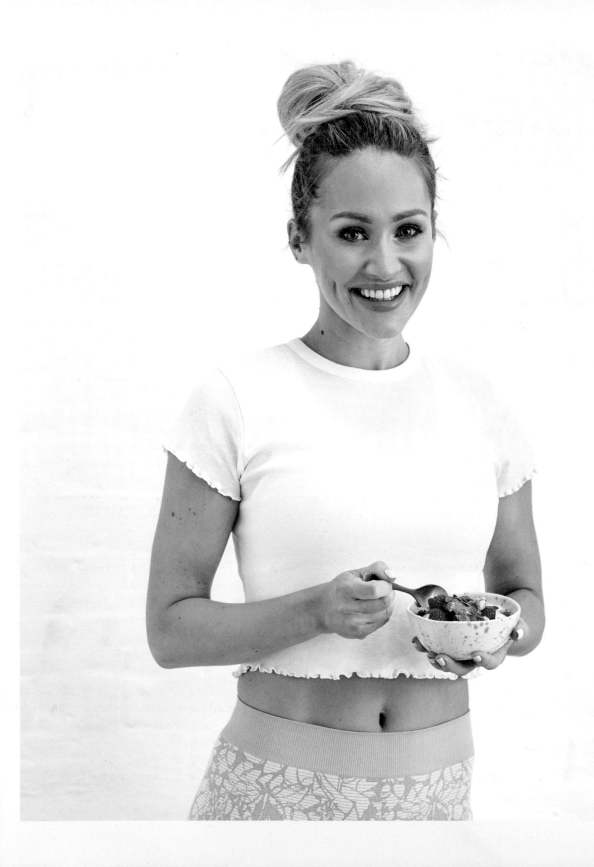

> I am really passionate about being myself because I know how it feels to struggle with self-worth

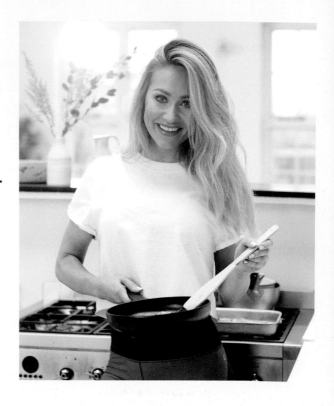

minutes (ahhhh, the dreaded bloat!) that I realised that sharing my day-to-day life was so much more real.

My bloating images gathered a lot of attention on social networks. I always try to be honest with people through what I post, as there are so many unnatural edited images that we see on a daily basis. I am really passionate about being myself because I know how it feels to struggle with self-worth, body image and just generally being confident in your own skin. But still, I was amazed at the comments and messages from people all over the world who shared their stories with me and thanked me for comforting them so they didn't suffer alone. Along with the national media coverage of my bloat, it made me realise just how many of us suffer from conditions that result in extreme pain

and abdominal bloating and experience our symptoms alone, in silence.

Irritable bowel syndrome (IBS) is a chronic condition that affects the digestive system, and is a gastrointestinal disorder that I have had for most of my life. Symptoms include abdominal pain, bloating and increased gas – which we like to call sitting on a duck. There are different types of this disorder which can affect everyone in a variety of ways: constipation and diarrhoea are the most common, and for me it has been made worse because of my PCOS.

In addition, food intolerances and stress are all triggers that can affect your body and cause bloating, and I for one suffer from the majority, if not all, of them.

my lifestyle

I wasn't always the fit, healthy, happy person that I am so proud to be today. Five years ago, I was just a shadow of my current self, weighing a very worrying 46kg. Was I happy? Absolutely not! I was depressed, underweight and unhealthy. All my life I was told who I would be and what I should be. I read once that 'If conforming to everyone's expectation is your number one goal, then you have sacrificed your uniqueness and therefore your excellence'. Everything I tried to be for everyone else just made me feel limited; I lowered my expectations of myself and I felt less in control of who I was and wanted to be. I was trying to be perfect and I think I was just trying to be someone I am not.

As a former professional dancer and model, I have always been very competitive, but working in such cut-throat industries lead to me becoming obsessed with my weight and appearance. Trying to be perfect couldn't have made me any more unhappy. I had a poor diet, was doing too much cardio and I was constantly comparing myself to unrealistic images in magazines, online and on social media. 'I'm fine', was the most common lie I told. I always focused on the negative, and found that constantly critiquing myself was destructive to my confidence and self-esteem. I thought I was eating healthily when really I had no idea about nutrition. I always wanted to be thinner, and I felt fat even though everyone would tell me I was tiny. It was mentally and physically draining, a horrible way to live that I wouldn't wish upon anyone.

People often change when there is a traumatic life-altering event, and so it was for me. In 2015 I suffered the biggest heartbreak, after an amazing four-year relationship, overnight I lost my best friend. I had given myself in full to a person I adored and I got my heart back in a million pieces. It was in the process of fixing myself that I discovered who I really am. Self-love, self-respect, self-worth, there is a simple reason why you can't find them in anyone else. To love yourself, you must stop hating yourself for everything you are not and start loving yourself for everything that you already are.

So, I am super excited to share with you to how I live my daily life – my ups and downs, workout guides, secret remedies and daily recipes that I make time and time again. I lead a pretty hectic and busy lifestyle – who doesn't? Whether you're running around the city, looking after your family or travelling for work, we all have our own version of busy, and this book caters to every lifestyle. We are only human; we don't have to have it together every minute of every day. I am constantly on the go; some days I have no idea how I will get through everything, but every single day I just do it and if I don't have the right fuel to keep me going, well, hell hath no fury when I'm inconvenienced and 'HANGRY!'

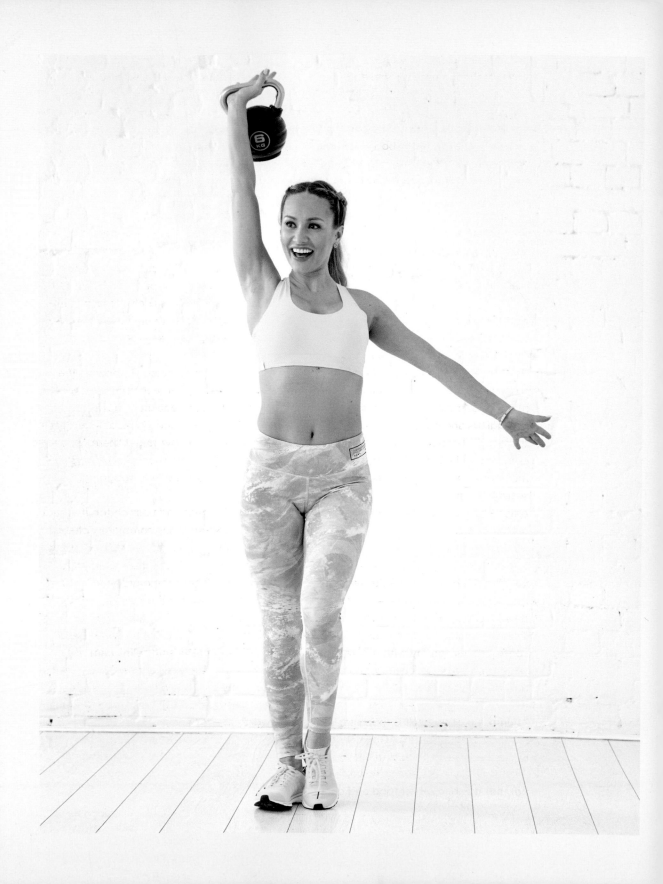

My aim is to keep every recipe in this book quick, tasty and easy for you and your loved ones. It is a collection of everything I do when I want to see real results and keep the bloat under control. Every effort – big or small – changes your body from the inside out. I want to empower women, so I've written this with that and their needs in mind so that they can create healthy habits, not restrictions. I love it when women love themselves and when they inspire other women to love themselves. Remember, the reason you are reading this guide is to make your life better.

Let's face it, abdominal bloating can make us look like we are pregnant. I feel like Regina George from *Mean Girls* half the time because sweat pants are all that fit me. Luckily, being in the fitness industry means that most of my wardrobe consists of leggings and sweat pants, but those crop tops – ugh, someone hand me a baggy t-shirt from the 90s! Bloating causes us so much physical discomfort, and it always seems to come at the most inconvenient of times – holidays, parties, family occasions or date nights!

So I'm going to guide you on how to beat your bloat, create new habits, and help prevent the bane of your life creeping up on you when you least expect it. But when it does, my guide will be your go-to for soothing your tummy with natural home remedies, relaxing yoga and delicious bloat-busting nutrition.

Taking care of yourself is much easier than you think; I want you to know that it is possible to live a fun, enjoyable and healthy lifestyle. It's not complicated, it's not about eating rabbit food and counting calories or macros, and it most definitely is not a constant battle with yourself and your mind. Becoming my version of fit and healthy has helped me immensely with my confidence. I'm living life to the best of my ability and I want you to feel this way too.

Not only will the food you eat make you look and feel awesome, but sleep, stress management, exercise, beauty and self-care all play a huge role in a healthy lifestyle. In fact, I consider it a full package and just as important as what I put in my body. I want to give you all the tools you need to get there, so you will not only hit your habit-changing goals, but completely change your lifestyle for the better.

I have been where you are now, at the starting point, where it all begins. You've taken this step because you want to change; the next step is reading and understanding how to get there. My secret is simple, if you're tired of starting over, stop giving up and let's get going.

The excitement and passion for life that I have discovered has completely changed me. I no longer stress about if I'm going to get bloated. Every morning I wake up excited about the day ahead, excited to train and excited to nourish my body with delicious healthy food so that it can function to the best of its ability. I am confident, I have self-belief, I am truly happy and I love myself for who I am. It's up to me to make my life the best life possible because, at last, I believe I am worth it!

my nutrition

My journey with food has been quite the rollercoaster, of intolerances, emotions, and bloat. I feel like I have majorly experimented, trying and testing every de-bloating method and finally found a balance. Nutrition is never about eating less, or low in calories. My nutrition doesn't leave me feeling hungry or tired because I believe that nutrition is about fuelling your body with real whole foods.

Some days I spring out of bed and feel like I can conquer the world, while on other days it takes me two hours just to peel back the duvet. I also suffer from adrenal fatigue, a condition that stops your adrenal gland, pituitary gland and hypothalamus functioning properly. Basically, your body slows down when under stress, so I feel like I need to sleep for three years and my digestive system, well, that's why we are here reading this.

My nutrition is almost always on point and I exercise daily, but my body just needs a little more rest than usual. When you suffer from conditions like IBS, SIBO or PCOS, these all cause the body quite a bit of stress, and alongside hormonal imbalances it can be common that you are not always absorbing all the nutrients from the foods you are eating. How do we establish the right hormonal balance? Getting a good night's sleep is key to keeping your hormones in check, and one of the best ways to balance your hormones is through diet. It is always best to get all your nutrients naturally through the foods you eat and not through supplementation.

Back to the big words. The hypothalamus (sounds like a dinosaur) is extremely important, kind of like the control centre of our hormones. It controls our emotions, weight regulation, sleep, when we feel hungry, thirsty and even our body temperature. When it's not functioning correctly, we don't function, hence the exhaustion. Adding the following foods to your diet can really help with the proper function of hypothalamus: turkey, green beans, oranges, sweet potatoes, basil, bananas, camu camu powder, spirulina, maca powder, salmon and eggs. The sources of anti-inflammatory, healthy fats that I find really work for me are olive oil, coconut oil, avocados and nuts. These foods help overcome adrenal fatigue because they're nutrient-dense, low in sugar and contain healthy fat and fibre.

Some days I spring out of bed and feel like I can conquer the world, while on others it takes me two hours to peel back the duvet

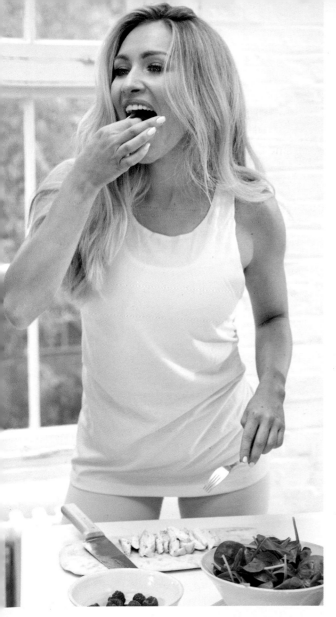

this is not a diet book

MAEVE: 'Warning, this book is NOT a diet book... YAAAS! Who has actually ever gone on a diet and survived? You: 'I'm on a diet, I really wanna lose 3lb, how hard can that be?' Fifteen minutes into the diet: 'I just want to eat everything, I want to eat 30lb of chocolate, I am in dieting hell!' We have all been there... FACT!

Beat Your Bloat is a simple guide to dealing with all the delightful female issues we have been gifted with (thank you, Eve) from PCOS to IBS and every other condition in between that has left us sucking in for dear life on many an occasion and night out.

HOW IT WORKS

My aim is that this book becomes your new best friend. I will be helping you find your own way towards leading a lifestyle that you love, building your confidence in being the best version of yourself and ultimately enabling you to find happiness and balance in all the new habits that you will be creating. It sounds 'fantabulous', doesn't it? All of these small changes add up to huge results. Start by sharing these on my forums and across social media, with me and everyone else beginning their journey. By supporting and encouraging each other, you are surrounding yourself with people who get it!

WHAT WILL I BE DOING?

It's time to get our excitamobility on. Setting small goals will scare you a little, but excite you a lot. No one wants to start off by climbing Mount Everest – that's impossible. With small changes, you will learn how to enjoy delicious, nutritious food for life, the secrets to controlling those outbursts of bloat, and fitting your fitness into a lifestyle that you love.

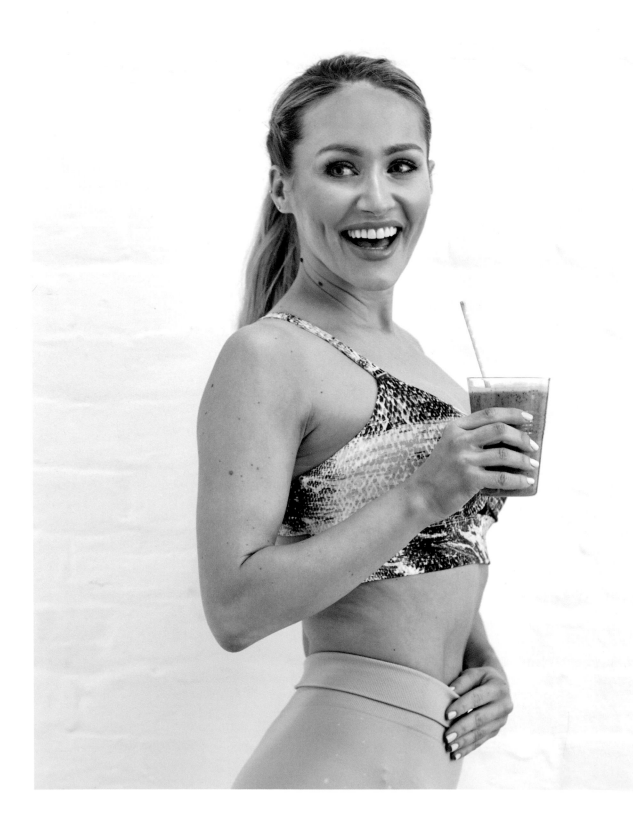

beating your bloat

food glorious food

I believe the most important thing about living a healthy, bloat-free lifestyle is that your food is always delicious, enjoyable and do-able. Nourishing your body with the right foods needs to fit into your lifestyle and not feel like a demotivating and irritating 'diet'. The worst word ever to exist is 'diet'. Any time I think or say that word I instantly feel like I have never been so hungry in my entire life and want to rush to the nearest junk-food store! Note to self: when I eat like c**p, I feel like c**p.

I like to eat four meals a day...Why? Because experience has taught me that if I eat less I find it hard to control my hunger. My sugar levels slump, I become very grumpy and more often than not this leads to binge-eating or grabbing some kind of sugary bar. Who knows if I'm actually crazy or if I just need some carbs in my life! If I know I'm eating several meals a day, though, I don't even think about snacking.

HAVE YOU THOUGHT ABOUT HOW YOU EAT? Your eating habits could be affecting your digestive system or be the very reason for your bloating. Knowing your relationship with food better and working out your weaknesses could show what's causing your bloat. Your gut is one of the best indicators of your overall health, also known as your second brain. Your gut can really guide you, and listening to your gut instinct could be your superpower.

If you eat cheese, drink milk or eat ice cream and you become gassy, bloated or feel sluggish, that's your gut talking to you. Listen to it, it's telling you something by causing an uncomfortable reaction. The pains you feel are messengers. Whatever you do, don't ignore your gut. Our digestive system is the foundation of our health, and self-care comes first.

Eating is such a vital part of our everyday lives, it literally keeps us alive and going strong. The nutrients we fuel our bodies with affect everything we do every day and how each cell functions. Of course, it will come as little surprise that how we eat and our relationship with food is very much a part of who we are and the type of person we are. So how should you be eating to avoid bloating? Simply, you should always be aiming to eat food in its most natural form. It's when you start to introduce 'fake', highly processed foods that you can begin to really struggle with gut issues.

WHAT TYPE OF EATER ARE YOU?

For many of us, our relationship with food is complicated. A rushed eater like myself, eating quickly and thoughtlessly on the go, usually struggles with IBS or SIBO symptoms. Not chewing your food properly causes bloating and indigestion; when you don't chew your food enough it's much harder for your body to break down the larger particles of food. So it's important to think about how you eat and identify what type of eater you are. Below are a few of the classic types – see which one looks most like you.

◆ **FUNCTIONAL EATER:** The functional eater is all about speed and convenience. They will have all the food-delivery apps downloaded on their phone, so they can access the quickest, most convenient way to get food.

◆ **EMOTIONAL EATER:** A true emotional eater won't think about the future consequences of what they are consuming. They are generally looking to satisfy an emotion with food – what and how they eat goes back to how they feel. Ironically, the emotional eater will eat foods that make their blood sugar to fluctuate, causing them to hop onto that rollercoaster of emotions.

◆ **BINGE EATER:** A binge is an episode of excessive, uncontrollable eating or drinking. People who binge eat very large quantities of food over a short period of time, even when they're not hungry.

◆ **YO-YO DIETER:** Yo-yo dieters are constantly either on a diet or off it. These diets are often extreme, so they lose a lot of weight. I think of yo-yo dieting as the tendency to be either 'all in' or 'all out' when it comes to weight loss. And, as your attention to nutrition goes up and down, so does your weight.

◆ **SECRET EATER:** The number of people who are eating in secret or hiding the food they are eating is startling. Many of us glory in eating healthily in public, but are piling in the junk food behind closed doors, gorging in the absence of other people and then shamefully hiding the evidence as if it didn't happen.

◆ **TASK SNACKER:** You almost always eat while doing something else, like watching TV, talking on the phone, answering emails, working at your desk or even cooking. It is a completely subconscious way of eating that can lead to overconsumption of food.

◆ **CONSTANT GRAZER:** The constant grazer will do exactly that. Instead of eating three meals and perhaps a snack throughout the day, the constant grazer will pick and nibble all day long.

◆ **DISTRACTED EATER:** You eat behind the wheel, at your desk or standing up in front of the fridge. This keeps you from concentrating on what you're eating and makes it more likely you'll overeat.

◆ **THE INSTAGRAMMER:** This is a new one – the camera eats first. No one touches anything until the perfect picture has been captured and then we wait another 20 minutes while we choose a filter to post the picture-perfect brunch, which in reality has really been a rather stressful and distracting experience!

CREATING GOOD FOOD HABITS

◆ Once you can identify your eating habits it makes it so much easier for you to write a meal plan that you can stick to using my recipes. So take a little time to think about how you approach food before you think about other factors in your diet, such as, should you be counting calories and macros? Personally I don't – instead I ask myself where the food came from and if it's nutritious. Nutrient-rich foods will keep you fuller for longer and help to maintain stable blood-sugar levels, which will minimise your cravings.

◆ Try to eat mindfully by making time to prepare fresh food that nourishes your body and satisfies your appetite. Eating mindfully means you set aside time for each meal to relax and focus on what you are eating rather than combining two or three tasks simultaneously – this is important for all types of eater, not just Task Snackers (see page 17).

◆ Hydration is key to a well-functioning digestive system. Being dehydrated can often lead us to eat the wrong foods and make us feel tired and sluggish, which in turn will lead you to reach for another cup of coffee and a possible side of sugar. The best and simplest way to hydrate our bodies is by drinking plenty of filtered water.

◆ If you are a snacker of unhealthy treats, a good way to avoid giving into your cravings is by detoxing your kitchen or your work environment of all the sugary stuff. Keep your home stocked with nourishing foods and prepare healthy snacks to keep at work so they are conveniently ready for you to eat. No matter how much you hide away sugary snacks, the moment you feel stressed or have an energy slump you will find yourself dragging a chair over to the high treat cupboard and indulging in a quick pick-me-up.

◆ A lot of us equate healthy food with tasteless, boring dishes. I recommend investing in some fun new kitchen utensils that will make cooking even more enjoyable. Who doesn't love a good spiraliser? It's like playing with Play-Doh as a kid, only this time you can actually eat the spaghetti!

◆ Making what we eat and how we prepare our food a priority is often quite strange for many of us. We seem to be able to schedule the gym, hang out with friends, watch every episode of our favourite series on Netflix into our daily life, but can't put enough time aside to consciously prepare and enjoy what we eat. Nourishing yourself is just as important as all the other things we do to improve our wellbeing. A healthy life starts from the inside out, so if we can fit in nail appointments, haircuts and facials, we can love ourselves enough to live well.

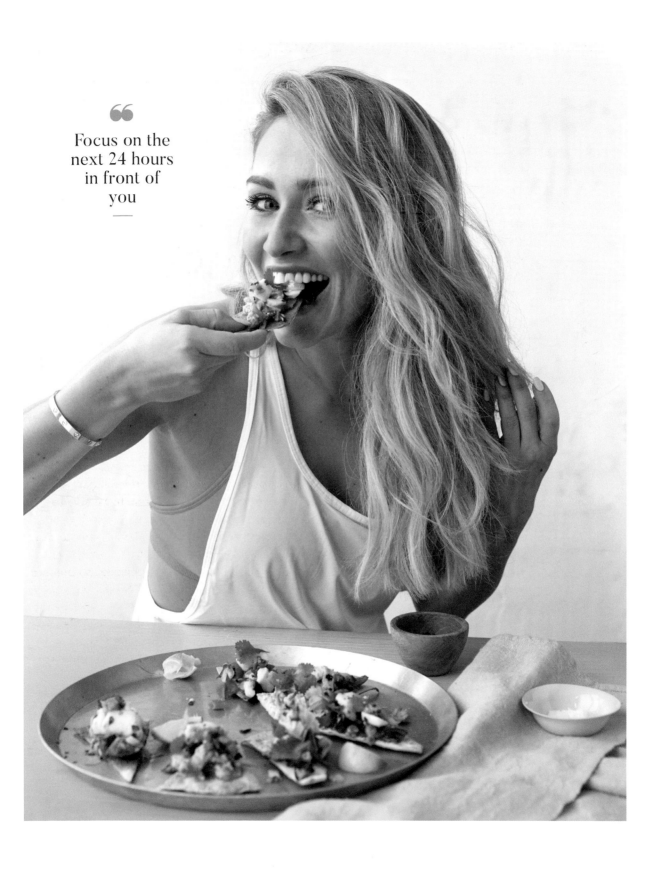

> **"**
> Focus on the
> next 24 hours
> in front of
> you
>
> —

cut the cravings

I know how difficult it is to get off the sugar and stay off it, even those of us with the strongest willpower can find it difficult to crush those cravings. Be realistic and remember a slip-up does not mean that you have failed. Our goal is to keep our blood sugar levels even. Try my smart sugar tips to help beat your cravings.

7 WAYS TO STOP CRAVINGS

◆ FIGHT IT

The little sugar gremlin that comes alive every night is so difficult to fight because our willpower depletes through out the day. Ever have the healthiest of days and come 10pm find yourself munching though almost everything like the very hungry caterpillar? Tell yourself, 'this is just the sugar monster' and have a large glass of water or maybe a flavoured tea and then wait for 15–20 minutes. Remember if it's late at night you are probably just sleepy so stop binge watching a series and get a good night's sleep

◆ GO WITH YOUR GUT

Munching on too much sugar does not only damage the digestive system, but destroys the good bacteria in our gut, which can leave us feeling sluggish with a depleted immune system. Eating too much sugar can leave our gut acidic and bloated. Reaching for a good probiotic or drinking my beat the bloat drink (page 35) containing apple cider vinegar can help break down candida overgrowth in the gut.

◆ SLEEP DEPRIVED

Prioritise your sleep and your cravings will soon balance themselves out. You should be getting at least eight hours of sleep every night, so stop watching just one more episode on Netflix and get to bed! I know it's easier said than done, but your body will thank you. So please trust me, not dreamy Michael Scofield (aka Wentworth Miller in *Prison Break*)...

◆ SNACK ATTACK

If you think you're really hungry and fancy a wee treat, even though you have eaten proper meals during the day, stop, go to the cupboard and get a handful of almonds or a few berries. If you don't want them and you're just looking for sugar, you're not really hungry.

◆ THERE'S NO SUCH THING AS BITE-SIZED

We have convinced ourselves that we need to be constantly snacking, and with such a vast variety of so-called 'healthy', snack-sized treats available in almost every store, we seem to be snacking a lot more than we need to be. What you don't buy you won't eat, so try to keep sweet, sugary foods out of the house – no matter what their size.

◆ FOOD IS FUEL

Snacking is simply for the moments when 'hanger' sets in. Let me simplify the word 'hangry'; (noun) a crazed state of anger caused by lack of food and a major slump in sugar levels, which results in a psychotic meltdown and major binge-eating. Remember, when your body is hungry it wants nutrients.

◆ JUST SAY NO!

Say NO to artificial sweeteners. In fact, I often find that faux sweeteners make me crave sugar even more. So ditch those diet drinks.

FOOD HABITS & MOOD DIARY

We have all had those moments where we look down and see we are surrounded by wrappers, wine glasses, empty takeaway cartons and think 'OMG, what the hell just happened?! How could I lose control like that?' Cue emotions of regret, shame, anger and sadness. It's an emotional rollercoaster – and I'm riding up front.

Most people think binge-eating is due to lack of self-control and discipline, but I don't believe this is true. My lifestyle, which I have shared with you on social media, is very much about control and discipline. Growing up as a competitive athlete and dancer I achieved my goals and success in both these careers, and if it was really that simple I don't think these epic meltdowns would consciously occur for me. So how have I learned to get off the rollercoaster?

One of the best ways to identify the patterns behind your eating is to keep track of them with a food and mood diary. If hunger is not the problem, eating is not the solution. Do you find yourself eating way more than your body needs, sometimes to the point where you are eating yourself into a food coma, feeling like you're going to explode? You can do it sometimes without even knowing it, because it has become a habit, and in some cases it can turn into a bingeing disorder.

Over-indulging can feel great for a moment until that sense of regret kicks in. Every time you overeat or feel compelled to reach for your version of comfort food (committing carbicide), take a moment to figure out what triggered the urge. If you backtrack, you'll usually find an upsetting event initiated that need to binge.

Binge-eating and overeating is letting us know that some part of our life needs deeper attention and care. It's time to break up with binge-eating for good. This could be the day you stop doing that self-destructive thing you do.

Write it all down in your food and mood diary: what you ate (or wanted to eat), what happened to upset you, how you felt before you ate, what you felt as you were eating, and how you felt afterwards. Over time, you'll see a pattern emerge. Downloadable diaries are available at www.maevemadden.com.

Over-indulging can feel great for a moment until that sense of regret kicks in

This very result that you can see in front of you may be upsetting, but each of us carries so much love in our heart, it's time to give that love to yourself. This can be the beginning of designing a life you love. How exciting!

The next time you feel the urge to binge, instead of giving in, take a moment to stop and investigate what's going on inside. Are you going to be happy with yourself when you eat this? Try to identify the emotion you are feeling. Have you had a bad day at work? Relationship problems? Studying for exams, feeling lonely, shame, anxiety, major PMS, lack of self-confidence? These emotions do not define who you are as a person, they are simply passing you by. Feel that feeling but do not become it, challenge yourself to control the way you respond to it.

You're much more likely to overeat if you have junk food, desserts and alcohol in the house. Remove the temptation by clearing out your fridge and cupboards of your favourite binge foods.

Stop restricting yourself. I know you're thinking, 'Maeve, are you crazy? Why would I eat more?' Well, as DJ Khalid would say, 'Major Key...' So let's start this idea with eating more of the right foods instead of the wrong foods. Combining healthy carbs and protein creates more of the 'happy' hormone serotonin in your body. Serotonin is our new best friend; when our serotonin is low we get that intense craving for sugary foods. The biggest producer of serotonin in the body is the gut, and when our gut is happy, we are happy. When you add more nutritious deliciousness to your plate you will naturally start removing the negative nasties and stabilising your blood-sugar levels, which are key here. When you are already full on the healthy, good-for-you foods, you won't find yourself craving sugary sins.

Exercise is the most potent and under utilised antidepressant – and it's free! Regular exercise helps to stimulate our good friend serotonin, and the natural endorphins we receive from exercise remain increased in our system long after we have crushed a workout. Remember, the reason you are doing this is to make your life better, you are working on yourself, for yourself, by yourself. That is pretty empowering.

Letting yourself get too hungry or too tired is the best way to hop on that rollercoaster of vulnerable emotional eating. Sleeping beauty certainly had the right idea. OK, maybe she had the worst sixteenth-birthday party ever, but getting plenty of sleep regulates how much leptin the body produces; leptin is the hormone that lets us know when we've had enough to eat and when we're full.

When our body is hungry or tired, it not only sends strong messages to our brain that encourage us to eat, but more often than not discipline and self-control go out of the window. Ever wonder why you're starving all day long when you are tired or have had a bad night's sleep? Major lack of sleep reduces our levels of leptin (our 'full' hormone) and when we don't have much leptin, the hunger pangs just keep coming so we don't know when we are full. Invest in your rest.

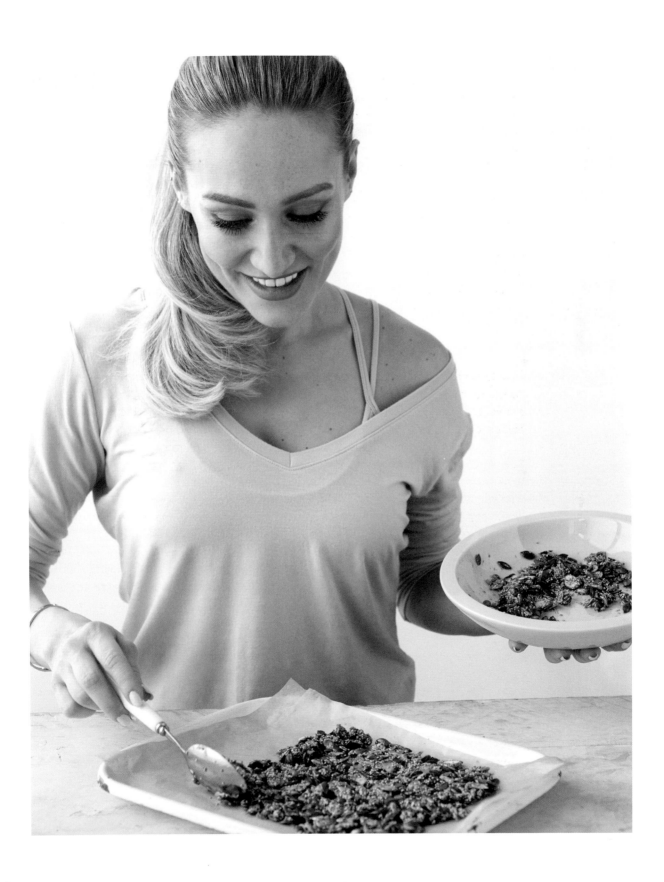

change a habit in 21 days...

It takes 21 days to create a habit. You will never change your life unless you change something you do daily, so the secret to creating new habits is to change your daily routine. The best project you are ever going to work on is you, so let's get started. (You can download a Change a Habit in 21 Days progress chart at www.maevemadden.com.)

Firstly, we are not going on a diet – they don't work anyway – so ditch the D word! We are getting ready to create a happy, sustainable lifestyle, one that is simple, quick and easy to maintain. You are going to transform your body and the way you eat, creating healthy habits, not restrictions. A little progress and a little change will add up to big results, I promise.

Everybody's lifestyle is different; some of us need more fuel than others, depending on our day-to-day demands. If you're training hard or have a very active lifestyle you're going to need more fuel than someone who sits at a desk or does little to no exercise. We all come in different shapes and sizes, so altering each recipe to meet your needs is highly recommended.

The most important thing to remember is never to go hungry – no one likes a 'hangry' diva anyway. When your body is hungry it wants nutrients, not calories, so pay close attention and make a note to yourself. If you're not hungry enough to eat a piece of fruit or veg, are you really that hungry?

Nutrition, fitness and mindfulness make a healthier, happier you. A happy mind leads to healthier eating, an energised body will inspire you to make better food choices to fuel those awesome workouts, and nutritious, delicious food heals and revitalises your body, making you healthy from the inside out.

A happy mind leads to healthier eating, and an energised body will inspire you to make better food choices to fuel those awesome workouts.

| PERFECT PROTEINS

Protein is part of just about every bodily function, and eating a diet rich in this macronutrient has a number of amazing health benefits. We need to eat protein every day to maintain our energy levels, stabilise blood sugar and support the absorption of nutrients. In fact, our hair and nails are made mostly of protein. Our bodies love protein as they use it to build and repair muscle and tissue, and since adding it to every meal I have reaped huge benefits – my hair is thicker, healthier and grows like no tomorrow. Don't worry if you are vegan or vegetarian, there are plenty of non-animal products that are high in protein to choose from in my recipes.

My favourite protein-rich foods are organic chicken, fish and eggs, which can be easily added to any breakfast, lunch or dinner recipes. I prefer to choose organic proteins where possible, as it ensures the animals were fed nutritious food with no additives, not pumped with antibiotics and other drugs, and were also able to roam outdoors and not spend their lives cooped up. Skinless chicken breasts, turkey, white fish and egg whites are the best sources of lean protein.

Black beans are another favourite. Although these little energy beans help cleanse our digestive tract, I try to limit my intake as legumes can cause gaseous explosions, leading to bloating. Black beans are an excellent source of both protein, and fibre, and are perfect for those following a vegan or vegetarian lifestyle.

| FABULOUS FATS

It still amazes me when I see friends or family reach for fat-free options in the supermarket. Most of these products have had all the good fats removed, but they are replaced with sugary carbs, artificial sweeteners and chemicals. These will spike your blood-sugar levels, leaving you even more hungry. Good, natural fats are fabulous, and you should include plenty of them in your diet to promote a gloriously healthy gut.

Good fats will give you youthful, glowing, plump skin and help you to keep your weight balanced and feel energised. Worried about choosing the right fats? My rule is, usually, if it comes from Mother Nature, it's good; if it comes from a factory and with a whole long list of unusual ingredients, it's bad. So get into the habit of checking the label.

I cook with healthy fats, using olive oil at lower temperatures but mainly in dressings, and I use avocado oil and coconut oil at higher temperatures. I avoid any kind of processed vegetable oil or palm oil. Fats are fab because they are our most powerful food energy source – more than protein and veg. They fill you up, so it's very hard to binge on good fats. But before you get too excited, keep in mind the difference between the good, the bad and the really freakin' awful (trans fats).

| CONSCIOUS CARBS

Carbs get a bad rap. Fad diets appear warning us to be conscious of carb intake and encouraging us to limit them, but we don't like the D word here. Good carbs are essential, helping us stay fuelled all day long. When we think of carbs we usually think of simple carbs like bread and pasta, but complex carbohydrates are contained in many of the foods we should be eating, including vegetables, fruits and grains like oats, brown rice and quinoa. These are packed with an abundant source of energy that our bodies need to function daily. So just as we shouldn't fear the fats, there are plenty of reasons to say yes to carbs.

Healthy food is happy food. Most people have no idea how amazing they will feel waking up each day by creating new healthy habits. Vowing to never eat a certain food again is just setting yourself up for failure. I can't swear that I will never ever eat another chocolate or drink a cocktail, and that kind of restriction more often than not just leaves me craving it even more.

A healthy lifestyle is all about balance; creating new, healthy, enjoyable habits, not restrictions. Each of us is perfectly imperfect in every way. I have provided you with recipes that you can mix and match to create your own day-to-day plan. I am here to guide you to beating your bloat with what has worked for me, and it could work so well for you, too. There is no one specific lifestyle plan that works miracles; our bodies are all uniquely individual and you need to discover what works for you so that every day you have the opportunity to wake up and work on being the very best version of yourself.

tips

◆ **Stay hydrated.** Drink as much still, filtered water as you can throughout the day. If you feel this is going to be a struggle, follow my recipe in the remedies section (pages 34–37).

◆ **Fuel your body** with 4–5 healthy, nutritious meals every day.

◆ **Be active for at least 30 minutes a day.** Start your week strong and finish your week stronger. Let exercise be your stress reliever, not food.

◆ **Start your day right.** Breakfast is the most important meal of the day and a healthy habit you want to keep for life. If you don't have time to wake up and make it, prep it the night before.

◆ **Invest in your rest.** Aim to get at least eight hours of sleep per night. Remember, the more tired you are the harder it is to resist temptation.

rescue remedies

There are so many causes of bloating. Need I remind you? OK! IBS, PCOS, PMS, SIBO, food intolerances, sleep deprivation and stress, to name a few. Thankfully, there are many home remedies that I have tried and tested that work, so I want to share these with you.

I also just want to give a big shout out to all the girls suffering with PCOS. I know just how hard it can be to live with this condition every single day, from the aches and pains to the emotional and physical distress. I never know what mood I'm going to wake up in. There is no cure and no explanation as to why we have it. We can only be brave and put a smile on our faces. I might act like it's not so much of a big deal, but really it can be emotionally heartbreaking.

While each of us is different, at some point most of us suffer from some form of tummy cramps. If you're bent in two with period pains, feeling insanely bloated (the damn bread basket) or suffering from IBS and trapped gas, ladies, these remedies can provide some relief.

YOGA

So, first up, whatever the cause, if you are stuck at home and all else has failed (it happens!), try my go-to home yoga workout, especially before bed.

Men, if you are reading this, don't worry, this is not a female-only yoga plan, you can join in, or skip ahead to the next page for other delightful home remedies.

So, get out the yoga mat and be ready to 'namaslay' or just get on the floor. Wear something comfy – Lululemon need not apply here, fluffy pyjamas are just as good. Don't worry, headstands and scorpion poses will not be included.

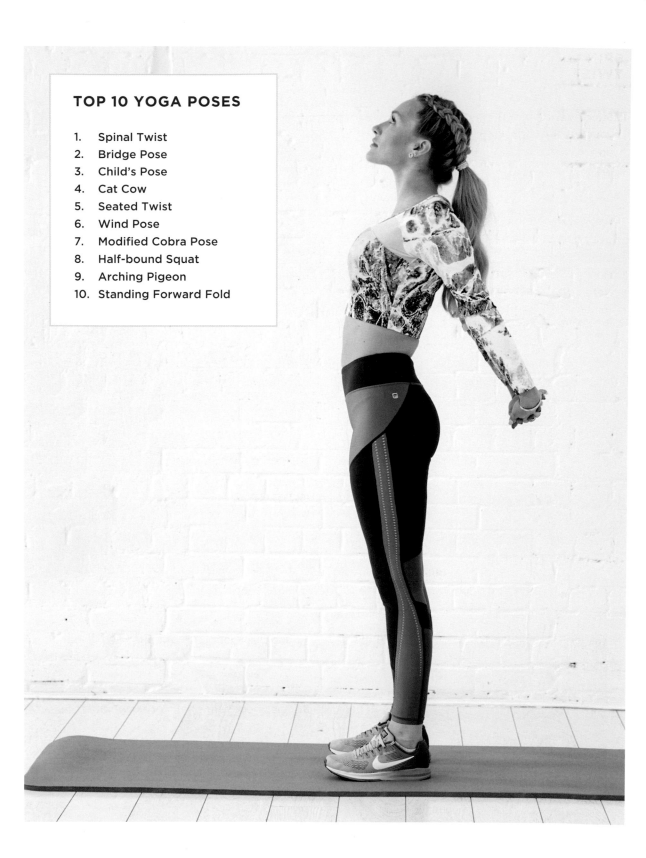

TOP 10 YOGA POSES

1. Spinal Twist
2. Bridge Pose
3. Child's Pose
4. Cat Cow
5. Seated Twist
6. Wind Pose
7. Modified Cobra Pose
8. Half-bound Squat
9. Arching Pigeon
10. Standing Forward Fold

SPINAL TWIST

1. Start by lying on your back with your knees bent and your feet flat on the floor. Your arms should be resting by your sides.

2. Drop your right knee to the floor and allow your left leg/knee to rest over the right leg.

3. Hold this position for 10–15 seconds. Return to the starting position and repeat on the opposite side.

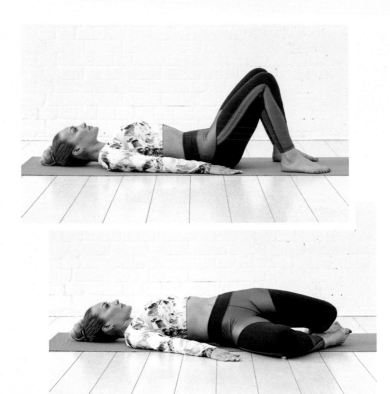

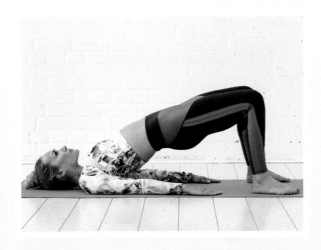

BRIDGE POSE

1. Start by lying on your back with your knees bent and your feet flat on the floor. Keep your feet hip-width apart.

2. Press your arms and feet firmly into the floor and push your hips upwards, raising your tailbone off the floor. Clench your bum while keeping your thighs and feet parallel.

3. Keep your hands flat on the floor and press your shoulders into the ground.

4. Lift your chin away from your sternum and then pull your sternum towards your chin to ensure a full stretch up through your back.

CHILD'S POSE

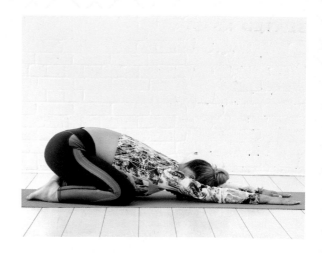

1. Start on your hands and knees. Push your knees wide apart with your big toes touching. Sit up straight and rest your bum on your heels. Stretch your spine and keep it straight.

2. Exhale and allow your body to drape between your thighs. Rest your chest on the top of your thighs and allow your head to touch the floor.

3. Extend your arms with your palms facing down. Push your hands slightly into the floor so that you are pushing your bum into your heels. Stretch through your hips and elongate through your arms.

4. Keep your lower back relaxed and make yourself as broad as possible. Try to avoid any tension through your shoulders, arms and neck.

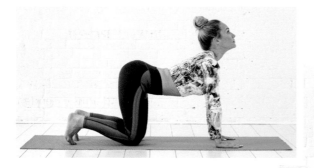

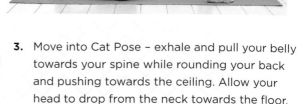

CAT COW

1. Start by kneeling on all fours with your hands directly under your shoulders and your knees and feet parallel to each other and hip-width apart. Keep your head centred and relaxed so that you
. are looking directly at the floor.

2. The first move is into Cow Pose – inhale as you lower your belly towards the floor. Your chin and chest should be lifted so that you are now looking towards the ceiling.

3. Move into Cat Pose – exhale and pull your belly towards your spine while rounding your back and pushing towards the ceiling. Allow your head to drop from the neck towards the floor.

4. Inhale as you move back into Cow Pose and exhale moving back into Cat Pose.

SEATED TWIST

1. Start by sitting with your back straight and legs extended out in front of you.

2. Bend your right knee and cross your right foot over your left leg so that it sits perpendicular to your left knee. Keep yourself balanced, elongate your spine and keep your neck relaxed.

3. Extend your right hand behind you and place it on the floor. Bring your left hand over your right knee. Exhale and twist gently to the right.

4. Inhale and straighten your back, then exhale and twist further. Repeat on the other side.
deeper twist. Hold for 10–15 seconds. Repeat the twist on the other side.

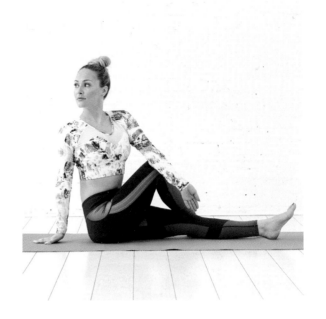

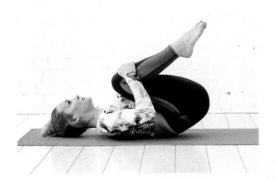

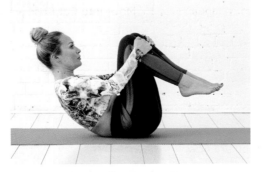

WIND POSE

1. Start by lying on your back, legs and arms extended as far as you can reach.

2. Exhale and bring both of your knees into your chest. Wrap your arms around them and clasp your hands together.

3. Rock backwards and forwards with your hands clasped around your knees.

MODIFIED COBRA POSE

1. Start by lying face-down on the floor with your legs extended and a couple of inches apart. Move your hands so that they are directly underneath your shoulders with your fingertips pointing forward. Your elbows should be tucked into the sides of your body.

2. Inhale, lift your head and chest off the floor, ensuring that your lower ribs maintain contact with the mat. Pull your shoulders back and your chestbone forward. Straighten your arms and lift your chest off the floor. This is Low Cobra.

3. Straighten your arms while ensuring that your pelvis keeps contact with the floor. This is High Cobra. Hold this position for up to 30 seconds. Exhale as you release and lower your chest towards the mat.

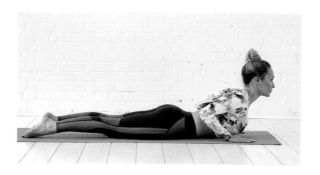

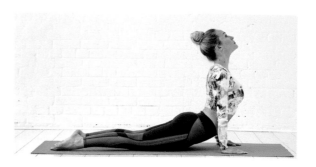

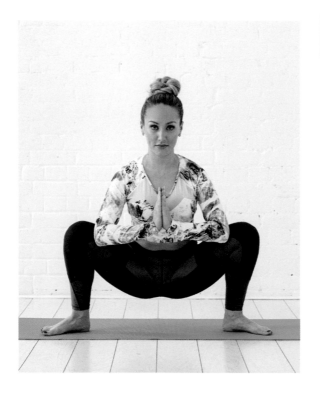

HALF-BOUND SQUAT

1. Start with your feet slightly more than shoulder-width apart. Point your feet outwards away from each other.

2. Bend your knees and lower yourself into a full squat position. Keep your core engaged and back straight.

3. Bring your hands together in front of you so that your elbows are touching your knees. Return to your starting position and repeat.

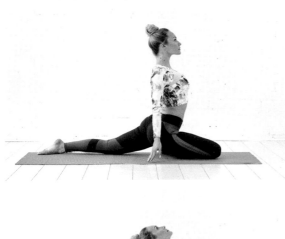

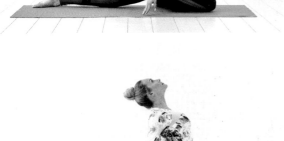

ARCHING PIGEON

1. Start on your hands and knees. Bring your right knee forward so your right foot is underneath your left hip and your left leg is extended behind you. Flatten the top of your left foot into the floor and sink your pelvis into the mat.

2. Slowly walk your hands back so that they are parallel to, or just behind, your hips. Ensure your head is centred directly above your pelvis. Draw your shoulder blades down and make yourself as broad as possible.

3. Extend your spine and pull your head and shoulders back. Your head should be extended back past your hips so that it is now parallel to your bum.

4. Hold the pose for 10–15 seconds and repeat on the other side.

STANDING FORWARD FOLD

1. Start by standing with your hands on your hips, feet slightly wider than shoulder-width apart.

2. While exhaling, bend forward from the hip joints, not from the waist.

3. Keep your knees straight, bring your palms (or fingertips) to the floor slightly in front of, or beside, your feet. Press your heels firmly into the floor while turning your thighs slightly inward.

4. While inhaling, lift and lengthen your torso. Then when exhaling, release further into the forward bend. Repeat the inhale and exhale 5–6 times while in the pose.

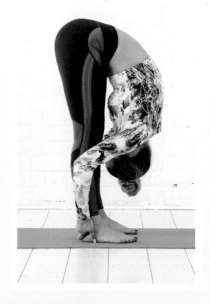

RESCUE REMEDIES

I know this is easier said than done, but do try to cut back on your sugar intake, especially during your period. You may think that sitting snuggled up with a hot water bottle on your tummy (that is recommended) and a big bar of chocolate and hot cuppa (not recommended) is what your body needs, but the sugar and caffeine in both are actually going to make your cramps so much worse. Ditch the chocolate, the caffeinated black tea and milk, which will send you on a sugar/mood spiral and leave you even more irritated and opt for something a lot more soothing.

'calm me' with camomile

serves 1

1 camomile tea bag
slice of apple or fresh ginger
½ teaspoon maple syrup

This drink will not only ease the pain but help to relax your body, so you can enjoy a great night's sleep, too.

Boil some water and add to a mug with the camomile tea bag. Add the slice of fresh apple or ginger along with the maple syrup. Stir.

sweet spicy saviour

serves 1

250ml almond milk or your favourite nut milk
1 tablespoon cacao powder
1 tablespoon vanilla extract
½ teaspoon ground cinnamon
¼ teaspoon ground turmeric
pinch of pink Himalayan salt
1 teaspoon maple syrup
1 teaspoon nut butter
crushed pistachio nuts, for topping

Turmeric is liquid gold and known for its amazing health benefits, especially for reducing inflammation and gut healing. I have used it in many of my rescue remedies, but this is the sweetest of all. I prefer to use almond milk here.

Combine all the ingredients in a saucepan over a medium–low heat. Stir frequently until the mixture is smooth. Pour into a mug and scatter some crushed pistachios on top for a little crunch.

tip Just ½ teaspoon of ground cinnamon is a fantastic anti-inflammatory and is known to stabilise blood-sugar levels, keeping those sweet cravings at bay.

my famous 'beat the bloat' drink

serves 2

2 tablespoons organic, raw apple
   cider vinegar
juice of 1 lemon
1 teaspoon ground cinnamon
3–4 ice cubes
1 teaspoon maple syrup (optional)

It spread across my social media and you have all shared your amazing photos when you have created my Beat the Bloat drink at home. I have added a little optional ingredient to sweeten it up, but for me this is my favourite remedy of all. I highly recommend apple cider vinegar as an aid to digestive stress and PCOS, but how to drink that foul-smelling liquid? I like to believe I have mastered it with this recipe!

Blitz all the ingredients together in a blender with 600ml water. Pour into glasses and drink immediately. (I highly recommend doing this through a straw to protect your teeth from the acidic vinegar.)

 tip Apple cider vinegar increases acid production, which may put excess stress on our body. Always remember to dilute apple cider vinegar with plenty of water.

mint choc-chip shake

serves 2

1 avocado, halved, stoned and
   flesh scooped out
250ml almond milk
a small handful of spinach
½ teaspoon vanilla extract
½ teaspoon cacao powder
1 drop peppermint extract or
   3–4 fresh mint leaves
½ teaspoon stevia
a handful of ice cubes

Yes, you read it right: a cool, fresh mint, chocolate-chip milkshake. This is one of my absolute favourite weekend smoothies – bloat or no bloat. Why peppermint? Well, peppermint works to calm the stomach muscles and improve bile flow, which the body uses to digest fats. This allows food to pass through the stomach quicker, aiding digestion and soothing stomach pains. Cacao helps the body produce endorphins, giving you that good-mood feeling.

Blitz all the ingredients together in a blender until smooth. Pour into glasses and serve immediately.

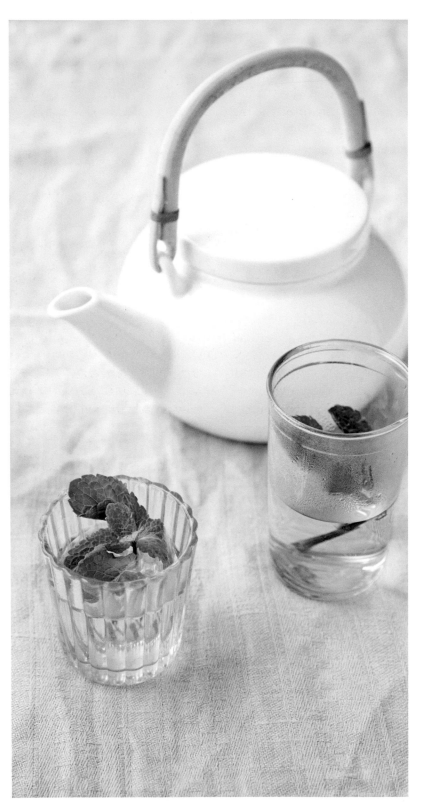

feeling fresh tea

Mint is a marvellous aid to digestion, I suppose that's why so many cultures have fresh mint tea after their meals. Mint contains a compound called menthol that aids in the normalisation of intestinal contractions. This is the perfect home remedy for anyone suffering with IBS. The natural oils found in mint help to break down and remove gas from the digestive tract.

Fresh mint leaves work well with both hot and cold water. This method is so simple. Place the leaves into an empty cup and add boiling water. Let it steep for 4–5 minutes before drinking. I like to remove the leaves before I drink the tea, otherwise you spend your time trying to avoid getting them in your mouth.

 tip You can often buy a mint plant at your local supermarket so that you always have leaves ready for a cuppa.

golden goddess milk

serves 2

300ml filtered water or
    almond milk
8 raw almonds
1 teaspoon turmeric juice
1 teaspoon ginger juice
½ teaspoon ground cinnamon
pinch of pink Himalayan salt
1 teaspoon maple syrup

If Cleopatra had the bloat, this would be what she would have drunk. Golden goddess milk is basically the Holy Grail of a beauty bloating drink, as the turmeric is an antioxidant and an anti-inflammatory blood purifier, which helps to relieve bloating and improve digestion.

Blitz all the ingredients together in a blender and watch it turn to liquid gold.

tummy tonic

serves 2

10 fresh mint leaves
1 teaspoon grated fresh ginger,
    or slices
1 lemon, finely sliced
½ cucumber, peeled and sliced

Hydration is key to avoiding water retention and aiding digestion. If you are suffering from constipation, headaches, burny pee, fatigue, dry skin or lips, the chances are you could be dehydrated. Water is an amazing source of energy as dehydration can cause us to feel tired and sluggish, so drink up.

I love drinking water, up to 3 litres per day, but I know many people do find it difficult to drink enough. Here is a quick, simple solution to getting in at least eight glasses per day, and it will also detox the body, helping keep you debloated. Making up a jug of this is a great way of measuring just how much water you drink throughout the day.

Put all the ingredients in a large jug or empty bottle with 2 litres of cold water. Stir to combine and leave to cool in the fridge for an hour or so.

tip

If you have yet to stock up on all the ingredients and create a Hogwarts-like cupboard for my potions, or you're still feeling exhausted or completely hormotional having taken an early vacation to menstrual island, don't worry, I have the answer. You are in need of a good home remedy now, so get ready for some serious r&r. Run a hot bath and add some Epsom salts or pink Himalayan salt. Sit in the bath and allow the salts to draw out the toxins, help to balance the hormones and leave you feeling relaxed and ready for a good night's sleep.

eating out & fast food

Ordering takeaways and eating out have very much become part of our daily lives. From breakfast meetings, brunch and lunch to catch-ups over coffee or cocktails, the list goes on. Most of our days, both spent socially or alone, revolve around food. I probably have at least one meal, snack or smoothie that I have NOT prepared at home every day. You can't control everything in your life, but you can control what you put in your body, so here are a few tips to help you to maintain those healthy intentions.

◆ SPEAK UP

Don't be afraid to tell your waiter before you order that you have a food intolerance or allergy. I used to be far too embarrassed to be open about my IBS, and like clockwork, minutes after eating, I would be guzzling fresh mint tea to try to calm my bloat. Be confident in your order, quiz your waiter about how the food is prepared and request something bespoke if you must. Remember, this is your time to relax and enjoy yourself.

◆ A LITTLE SIDE SAUCE

I once watched a chef pour an entire soup ladle of sauce over my food. To avoid this calorific, unnecessary overindulgence, ask for dressings and sauces on the side. You get to control just how much you want to add to get the precise flavour you like.

◆ FABULOUS FISH

There is nothing more delicious than fresh seafood and fish, and while there is no such thing as a perfect food, low-calorie and high-protein fish and seafood certainly come close to fitting the bill. Raw, steamed, grilled or baked are the safe words here; avoid anything pan-fried, fried, crispy, crunchy or sautéed as it will usually contain more fat and more cooking oils, which can trigger bloating.

◆ AVOID THE BLOAT BASKET

I love the smell of freshly baked bread, but my body does not love the reaction I get when I eat it. I automatically tell the waiter when I am seated that we won't be needing a bread basket, much to the delight of everyone I'm with... sorry, guys!

◆ DOGGY BAG

Think in terms of having a quality dining experience and not paying to fill your stomach to the point of bursting. If you're feeling full and you've still got food on your plate, you can always ask for a doggy bag and take the leftovers home to enjoy for lunch the next day.

◆ POP, CLINK, FIZZ

Steer clear of fizzy drinks – even the 'diet' options. The chemicals they contain, such as aspartame and sucralose, raise blood-sugar levels and affect the good bacteria in your gut. They can also make you feel bloated and even more hungry helping your willpower go out the window.

my tips for travelling

We have all been there, arriving at a glorious destination feeling bloated, gassy and wondering where the abtastic beach body we worked so hard for went! Firstly, you have a body and you're going to the beach, so embrace it, feel confident and fabulous because unless you're some kind of Victoria's Secret angel or a saint, the chances are you will get a little bloated. It happens to us all.

Holidays are one of the best ways of connecting with loved ones, having fun with friends and just letting go. Remember, don't beat yourself up so much; if you stress about it, it will only make things worse; this is your time to enjoy and relax! I know how it feels to be in pain, bloated, suffering with fatigue and trying to find that one floaty outfit that will hopefully fit. The good news is that you can have fun, indulge and hopefully the only stress will be how to control the humidity frizz volume of your hair. (That's one issue I have yet to master.)

Long-haul flights can be the start of your bloat. It's so uncomfortable for your digestive system – sitting for hours, eating and drinking, usually just out of boredom – and I feel like the cabin pressure just pumps my tummy full of gas. Thank goodness this can be somewhat avoidable.

Due to the lack of humidity on the plane, you are more likely to become dehydrated, so although that mini bottle of wine is tempting, try to stock up on a few large bottles of water before boarding. There's plenty of time for a cocktail when you

land. You may feel like that annoying person running in and out to the toilet, but, if it beats the bloat, pee freely.

Long-haul flights can be the start of your bloat. It's so uncomfortable for your digestive system – sitting for hours, eating and drinking

Plane food is, unfortunately, quite often packed with additives, sodium and carbohydrates. So pack your own snacks. Most airports now have many healthy options to choose from. Stock up on salad boxes, protein pots and packets of nuts – these are my on-flight go-to basics. Remember, your gut is super sensitive, so stick to foods you would normally eat on a day-to-day basis and hydrate yourself well.

My number-one tip when travelling is hydration. If visiting a hot destination, you need to almost double your usual water intake. Water will not make you bloated, but water retention will. Why does your body hold on to water? Because it is dehydrated. Instead of reaching for an ice-cold fizzy drink, which won't quench your thirst and may make you gassy, keep drinking water. Also, being dehydrated can make you overeat because your body thinks it is hungry when really you are just thirsty. I know a lot of people find drinking enough water difficult, so try adding some

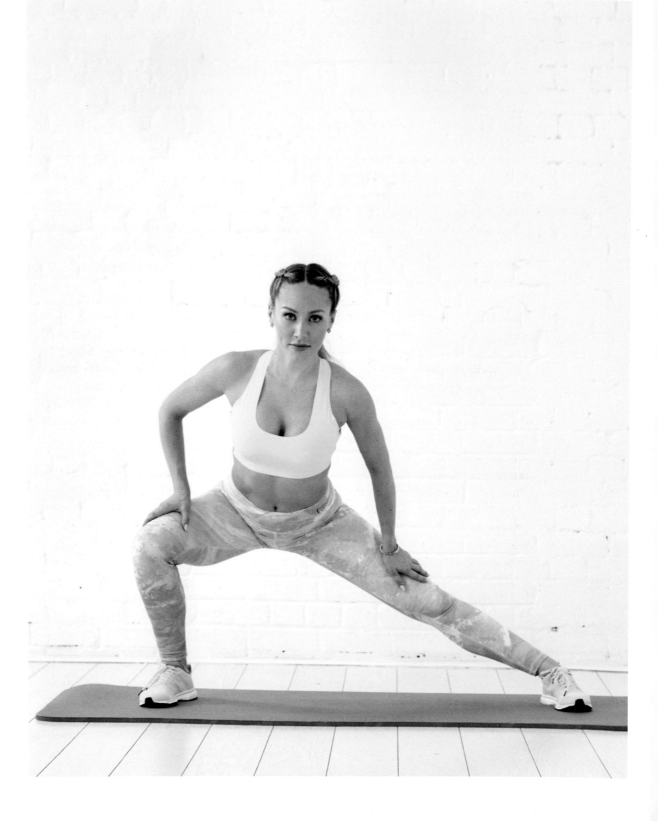

fresh lemon or lime to it. This will not only keep you hydrated, but will also help flush out the toxins.

Don't skip the sweat. Keep moving. One of the main reasons your system slows down on holiday is because you become more physically sluggish. Think about it: you probably sleep, then hit the pool or beach, where you sit around all day eating and drinking and then have a nap, followed by dinner and possibly dancing the night away before sleeping some more. Exercise and movement of any kind will help keep your bowels stimulated. Aim for 30 minutes of movement every day. If there is a hotel gym, hit it. You will enjoy the endorphins boost and feel bloat-free and awesome afterwards.

Try surfing, scuba diving or do some laps in the pool. Most holiday destinations have lots of outdoor sports on offer, so give them a go; plenty of Insta opportunities there! Hit up one of my home Instagram workouts or routines from this book in the room before heading out. I even have some holiday debloating 15-minute routines online, so you really have no excuses now.

If extreme sports are not your thing, a 30-minute walk along the beach will be enough. Walking barefoot in the sand can burn twice as many calories. It's not only healthy, but it exfoliates your feet at the same time – hello free pedicure!

Travelling abroad can be daunting when you have a sensitive gut and you're not sure what to eat. Firstly, let's not go mad on that holiday breakfast. It's so difficult to resist the temptation of freshly baked pastries, but our tummy doesn't know we are about to step into a bikini, so try to stick to the foods that you would eat at home. I try to have a high-protein breakfast, which helps to keep me fuller for longer.

Can we indulge without the bulge? The key to bloat damage control is to avoid the foods that you know will make you swell. I know and you know that eating that margherita pizza is going to end in swollen tears, and those salt-soaked cured meats have water retention written all over them. Think of the clothes you have packed. Avoiding starchy carbs, high-sodium and fatty foods is best, and I even avoid eating too much fruit, although it can be tempting, as fruits are high in fructans and can cause quite the swell. If you have travelled to a beach location, embrace the local culture, go Mediterranean and enjoy freshly caught fish, sardines, tuna or shellfish, which are all packed with protein and rich in omega-3, which encourages healthy digestion.

But let's be realistic here, too. You're on holiday, so if you do drink alcohol there is almost a 100 per cent chance you will be drinking and partying. Avoid champagne, if you can – alcohol is a bloater on its own, but adding extra bubbles takes it to a whole new level. If you are drinking, it's better to have spirits. Avoid high-sugar fruit juices and those highly calorific cocktails and beers. Always keep a fresh bottle of water on the table or with you to counteract the effects of water retention, stay hydrated and drink responsibly.

Most importantly, don't beat yourself up, enjoy the vitamin 'sea', relax, unwind and get into that flip-flop state of mind.

eat this, not that

Trust me, these smart food swaps can pave the way to a happier, healthier life. There are no excuses when it comes to making healthier food choices. Each small change to your lifestyle is an achievable way of reaching your goals.

Food sensitivities are the root of many of our health issues. Dairy can be the Darth Vadar and gluten the Godzilla of our most common gut problems. Never discredit your gut instinct; when something feels off, it usually is. Since our gut is the Da Vinci Code of our overall health, your reaction to either of these or other foods may not manifest in your gut but in other ways that you may not have suspected. Skin, moods, muscle and joint pain, fatigue or respiratory issues, to name a few. So you may be pleasantly surprised how you feel after a few days of these food swaps.

◆ ONIONS

Onions are one of my biggest bloating triggers. For me, onion is the most critical ingredient to find an alternative for as it seems to be in every recipe. I have completely cut out onion from my diet – and that includes white, red and brown onions, shallots and the white part of spring/salad onions and leeks. There are so many recipes, especially dinners, that include onion, so how do you get the same flavour? Although the white part of spring onions and leeks are best avoided, you might still be able to eat the green tops of both. These provide a super oniony flavour and can also replace white onions in some recipes, although I don't use onion in many of my recipes. Onion oil (who knew there was such a thing?) is a handy way of adding that oniony flavour. This works because onions are not soluble in oil, only in water.

◆ GLUTEN AND GRAINS

Grains containing gluten also happen to have high amounts of fructans, which consist of soluble fibre – a major no-no for the bloat. When fructans are fermented by gut bacteria they can cause gas, bloating and unusual bowel movements. I have been following a gluten-free lifestyle for quite some time now, and while luckily there are many gluten-free alternatives available, many of these are highly processed, so you need to be careful.

Gluten grains include wheat, spelt, rye and barley, as well as products made using these grains. Ever have a wheat breakfast cereal and end up feeling like Godzilla all morning? Never fear, the bloat boss is here! I recommended switching these grains for gluten-free oats, white and brown rice and quinoa. Yes, that means sushi is still on the menu for nights out. Italian food, on the

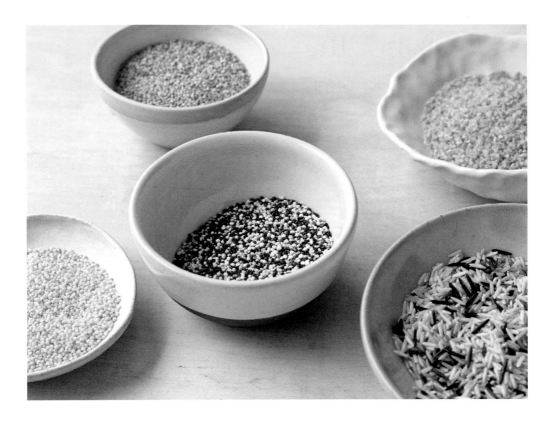

other hand, is a little more tricky. If you are a pasta lover, rice noodles or quinoa are generally good alternatives.

Sweet potato is also one of my favourite ways of replacing grains when you need something that's easy to make and a food that everyone enjoys.

◆ BREAD!

Wraps, pizza, sandwiches, croissants, soda bread and the like are all made with bloating bellyache ingredients. To be honest, bread is usually like that bad ex-boyfriend – we like it, but we really are not getting anything good from it. Commercially produced bread has little-to-no nutritional value and it makes us sad when we eat too much of it. Bread, like our exes, makes us feel good for an hour or so as it impacts our sugar levels. When you eat bread or any processed carbs, your blood sugar spikes and insulin level surges, you feel awesome, but not for long, because soon your blood sugar crashes and you feel like taking an afternoon nap, so you reach for more carbs to get that rush again. It's a vicious cycle. It's time to dump the bread – your gut knows what's up, so trust it.

What will you do without bread? OMG, the dilemma – it's like a little part of your life is over. No, not true, you're moving on to a better, bloat-free life.

I was introduced to collard greens, including kale and cabbage, during a summer trip to LA and at first I thought it was a bit of pretentious LA hipster food, but then I realised how awesome they are. Not only do they taste yummy but they are also super sturdy; so sturdy, in fact, that you can make a damn good burrito with them.

Rice wraps or rice cakes are one of my mother's staple swaps – I feel like our house in Ireland is full of rice cakes – but these delicious crunchy cakes are perfect for topping with tasty sandwich fillings – my Eggocado recipe (page 61) goes perfectly with them.

◆ DAIRY

Dairy is my arch enemy, not only does it make me bloat so it looks like I'm pregnant with a small elephant, but it makes me physically sick as well. My functional medicine doctor told me that if you get little bumps or red marks on the backs of your arm (the triceps) that could mean, and more than likely does mean, that you have an intolerance or sensitivity to lactose.

Dairy was once one of my favourite food groups – butter, ice cream, skinny milk cappuccinos, cheese – I consumed it on a daily basis. However, I have been lactose-free for about two years now and more often than not the smell of dairy makes me quite nauseous. Except for gelato – I still find it hard to resist that temptation.

Dairy isn't well tolerated by those who have IBS or SIBO, but also for quite a large number of us it's the lactose in dairy that's the brutal bloater. Adopting a dairy-free lifestyle is the best way to prevent any unwanted symptoms. All vegan recipes are marked with a 'V' symbol throughout.

Non-dairy alternatives are not as bad as you may fear. I can't have my oats without a little milk, and every now and then I still want to watch Netflix and chill with a bowl of ice cream. And, of course, I do indulge in chocolate, too. Almond milk, coconut milk, hemp milk and rice milk are all delicious milk alternatives that you can use, but do read the ingredients list on the packaging before buying as some brands do fill these with sugars, emulsifiers and other chemical preservatives.

Try to avoid oat milk and soy milk. One major disadvantage of soybeans is that they are high in phytic acid. What is that? It's a nasty substance that blocks your intake of essential minerals such as calcium, magnesium, iron and especially zinc, in the intestinal tract. I personally find it best to avoid any soy products.

Brown rice vs quinoa: Both are simple natural foods and easy to prepare. Quinoa is packed full of essential amino acids and has more protein than any other grain. If your protein needs are high or you are following a vegetarian or vegan lifestyle and not getting protein from meat products, eating more quinoa will provide a complete protein on its own.

EAT THIS!		NOT THAT!
Plain oats	◆	Sweet granola
Ground cinnamon	◆	Sugary topping
Nut milk	◆	Cow's milk
Almond butter	◆	Sugary peanut butter
Brown rice	◆	White rice
Sweet potato	◆	Potato
Almond butter fudge (page 126)	◆	Sweets
Nut butters	◆	Jam and chocolate spreads
Coconut yogurt	◆	Yogurt
Quinoa	◆	Couscous
Black Americano (with almond milk)	◆	Café latte
Water infused with fruit	◆	Sodas/Fizzy drinks
Stevia	◆	White sugar
Dark chocolate (approx. 70 per cent cocoa solids)	◆	Milk chocolate
Berries and coconut cream (see page 124)	◆	Strawberries and cream
Avocado	◆	Butter
Crudités	◆	Breadsticks
Spinach	◆	Iceberg lettuce
Sweet potato wedges	◆	French fries
Coconut oil	◆	Vegetable cooking fats/oils
Mashed avocado	◆	Mayonnaise
Avocado dressing	◆	Ready-made salad dressing
Himalayan salt	◆	Table salt
Quinoa	◆	Pasta
Grilled fish	◆	Fried fish
Vegan protein shakes	◆	Milkshakes
Dairy-free ice cream	◆	Ice cream
Unsalted nuts	◆	Crisps
Herbal teas	◆	Black tea
Air-popped popcorn	◆	Crisps
Vegetable juice	◆	Fruit juice
Poached/boiled eggs	◆	Fried eggs
Fresh fish	◆	Tinned fish
Roasted almonds	◆	Salted peanuts
Olive oil	◆	Butter
Green part of spring onions	◆	Red onion
Maple syrup	◆	Honey/agave
Blueberries	◆	Blackberries
Feta or Swiss cheese	◆	Cheddar cheese
Rice cakes	◆	Bread
Corn wraps	◆	Wheat wraps
Kiwi fruit	◆	Apples
Papaya	◆	Watermelon
Corn chips	◆	Nachos

confidence & monthly goals

THE RULES OF CONFIDENCE

Everybody is totally unique in their own special way. There is no one perfect body, because perfect does not exist. I know that living in our social-media-driven society can become a toxic mirror, as we are bombarded with the illusion of perfect bodies on a daily basis.

No matter your size or weight goals, let's shift the focus from body perfection and wanting to lose weight and be thin to self-acceptance and wanting to be stronger, healthier versions of ourselves.

It comes down to one simple question: if you don't believe in yourself, how do you expect anyone else to?

Get ready to bring on the feelgood vibes. I believe in you.

These are some of my body confidence tips that have helped me overcome my insecurities about who I wanted to be and instead accept who I am.

Confidence isn't bursting into a room with your head held high in some kind of fashionista diva style, thinking you're better than everyone else. Anyone who does that is probably lacking in self-confidence. For me, confidence is being happy and content in your own skin and not having to compare yourself to anyone. Self-confidence is the best outfit you can own.

When you catch yourself looking at yourself in the mirror, stop; don't be negative and pick out every single flaw. Know yourself and accept who you are. Pay yourself a compliment and tell yourself that you're beautiful. When you carry yourself with confidence you will naturally feel happy and more positive.

Stop comparing yourself to others and wishing you were something that you are not – we are all uniquely flawsome, we have our own strengths and weaknesses, and when you embrace who you are and realise you are enough, the magic starts to happen.

Your self-worth is not based on what you weigh, how many followers you have or how you look; you are enough. Always remember that just because you have had a bad day it does not mean that you have a bad life. Surround yourself with people who love and support you for being just the way you are. Be mindful and appreciate all that you have to be grateful for, write it down and remind yourself every day. This is your life and your story – only you can write it.

superfoods

You can't control everything in your life, and that's just nature, but you can control what you put into your body and how you choose to fuel your day-to-day life. We react to everything we eat: when we eat like crap, we feel like crap, but when we eat to nourish our bodies, that's when we flourish.

Good nutrition isn't low-fat, carb-free, sugar-free, or about eating just vegetables, feeling deprived and hungry. For me, good nutrition is about feeling fully energised, fuelling my body with all the nutrients it needs to feel healthy and happy, both inside and out.

But I don't just want to feel healthy, I want to feel awesome, and these are the superfoods you'll find in my cupboard of wonders that make me feel just that.

Why are these foods super? Well, they are the foods that contain a significantly higher quality of antioxidants, vitamins and minerals than any others. They are the Hollywood superstars of foods. Anti-ageing, bloat-beating, energising, disease-fighting. Not all of them are the weird and wonderful pulverised teaspoons of nutrition I have added to many of my smoothies and recipes, but some of these Oscar-winning superstars are everyday wholesome delights you find stocked on shelves at your local shops. Think blueberries, sweet potatoes, avocados, almonds, salmon and spinach, not just the more exotic superfoods grown in the rainforests of South America picked by handsome Amazonian Joe Mangellio-like warriors that send our nutritional daily

intakes soaring. OK, maybe I got a little carried away, but we can dream...

◆ **CAMU CAMU POWDER:** This powder is one of the greatest sources of acne-curing vitamins. One teaspoon is packed with 1,180 per cent of your recommended daily intake of vitamin C. Our skin is a great reflector of what is going on in our bodies – our stress levels, hormonal imbalances, diet and any intolerances all show on our skin. As a sufferer of hormonal acne outbreaks, I know how stressed and self-conscious you can feel living with this condition. Vitamin C is the mortal enemy of the stress hormone known as cortisol. If you are stressed out, your cortisol levels will be soaring and your skin can be more oily. Vitamin C is the warrior of vitamins, helping to diminish excess levels of cortisol, fighting acne and internal inflammation. It is also beneficial for reducing anxiety and boosting the immune system.

◆ **SPIRULINA:** The stimulator of good gut bacteria. Enough said. Just kidding. Don't be put off by the smell of pond when you open the packet (I've disguised the taste in my recipes). Why do we want to add this pond-tasting algae to our diet? Protein-rich spirulina boosts the body's ability to

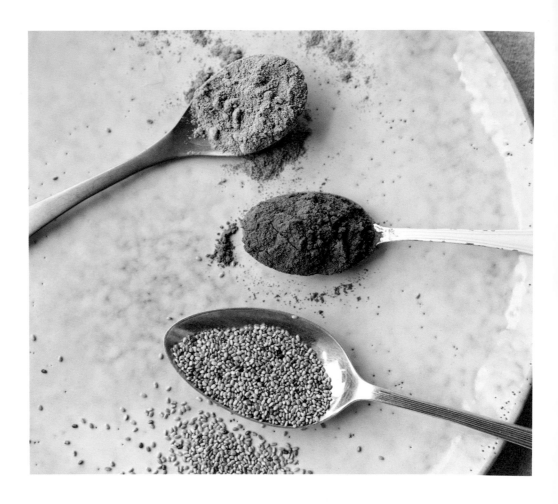

absorb nutrients and supports the growth of healthy bacterial flora in the gut, which can keep candida overgrowth at bay. It is packed with antioxidants and vitamin B, which is necessary for the digestion of fats and proteins.

Spirulina is one of nature's most potent nutrient sources. Thanks, Mother Nature. Not only is it good for our gut but our skin and hair, too. When I said that superfoods have a significantly higher level of vitamins and antioxidants, spirulina is pretty much at the top, winning all the Oscars and possibly an Olympic medal, too. It boasts healthy fats, a high content of amino acids, iron, zinc, copper, manganese, calcium and vitamins including A, C, E, K and B1, B2, B3, B5, B6 and B9 – all of which are essential compounds for clear, glowing, youthful skin and strong healthy, shiny hair. Who cares what it smells like now?! Luckily this beauty nutrient is available in pill, flake or powder form, so if the taste does throw you off, go for a high-quality capsule. The powder is easiest to use if you are blending it into smoothies (see First Aid on page 145). When choosing spirulina, try to buy one that is organic.

◆ **MACA:** While maca is good for both women and men, the benefits for women are substantial. Hormonal imbalance, PCOS, PMS, menopause and low libido are just a few reasons why you should introduce this into your diet. But what exactly is maca root powder? Maca is a great source of several important vitamins and minerals that boost energy levels and even enhance athletic performance. It is easy to incorporate into your diet as it can be taken as a supplement or added to smoothies, as I do, breakfast oats, and even baking.

I started using maca powder after being recommended it to help with hormonal imbalance. Having PCOS affects women differently. Some symptoms include weight gain, irregular or no periods, hair growth, acne and moodiness, and many of these symptoms are attributable to oestrogen dominance. Maca is believed to help by controlling oestrogen levels in the body. Having balance in the body and boosting our immune system is important for our reproductive health and alleviating all those nasty symptoms that we get from PCOS.

Using this potassium-rich supplement regularly provides a great boost of energy, more so than I gain from any kind of caffeine. I find one of the most positive aspects of using maca is the effect it has on my mood and my increased levels of energy. Having adrenal fatigue, I find I can get really tired and anxious, especially on the busiest of days. I say step aside coffee, this is a job for maca.

Your lifestyle is the sum of the choices you make, and the better the choices, the happier you will be. For every minute when we are moody, we lose 60 seconds of happiness. Maca me happy…!

◆ **BEE POLLEN:** Bee pollen contains enormous amounts of essential vitamins, minerals and amino acids. It helps to nourish every cell in your body, aiding digestion, increasing your metabolism, regulating bowel and intestinal function, boosting and strengthening your body and its nervous system. This makes bee pollen one of nature's best stress relievers. A little does go a long way, so we only need to add one teaspoon of nature's gold to our daily routine.

SUPPLEMENTS

Calcium, magnesium, selenium and zinc are some of the minerals that help with the symptoms of IBS and promote healthy digestion. I don't eat much dairy so I use a natural mineral supplement called Cellnutrition to ensure I consume some every day. I take hypertonic in the morning and an isotonic in the evening. As the hypertonic is bioavailable, the micronutrients work at a cellular level. This helps reduce inflammation in the bowel, soothing most of my symptoms of IBS. I always take one or two ampules prior to a night out as alcohol often flares up my IBS and there is no worse feeling than being bloated when I'm out.

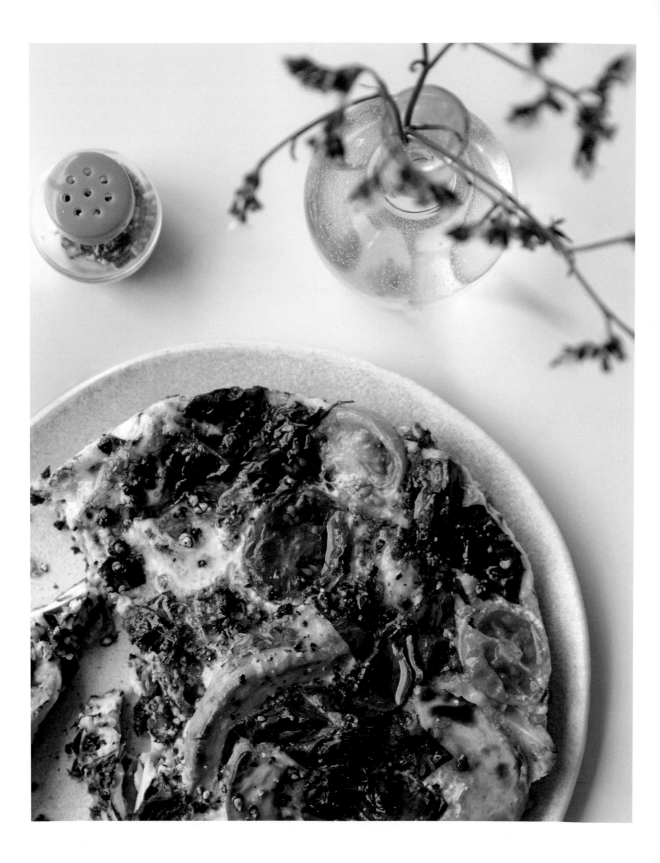

breakfast

happy huevos

229 CALORIES / 7G CARBS / 15G FAT / 18G PROTEIN

The typical huevos dish can be somewhat greasy and cheesy, and there isn't really anything happy about it. That's not the bloat-free morning we are looking for.

So get your mouth ready for a little morning fiesta, with four happy huevos. We are going to ditch the cheese and grease and fill our plates with nutritious deliciousness. Olé! Do you know how incredibly amazing a runny yolk tastes when combined with avocado, tomato, pepper and coriander? Let's find out.

serves 4

a handful of kale (about 30g),
   finely chopped
1 green pepper, deseeded and
   diced
1 red pepper, deseeded and diced
1 courgette, diced
4 tomatoes, diced
a handful of cherry tomatoes on
the vine
1 small red chilli, finely
   chopped
1 tablespoon olive oil
½ teaspoon coconut oil
8 eggs
salt and freshly ground black
   pepper, to taste
a handful of coriander leaves,
   to serve
4 lime wedges, to serve

Combine all the vegetables and chilli in a large mixing bowl. Season with salt and black pepper.

Heat the olive oil in a medium frying pan over a medium heat. Add one-quarter of the vegetable mix and cook, stirring, until warm. Make two holes in the middle of them in the pan and add the coconut oil. Crack two eggs, or one egg and one egg white, into the holes. Place the lid over the pan and cook for 4–5 minutes, or until the eggs are cooked to your liking.

Repeat this three more times for your breakfast buddies. Serve the salsa and eggs scattered with coriander and a lime wedge for squeezing over the top.

tip Add some gluten-free bread or wheat-free tortillas if you want a more substantial breakfast.

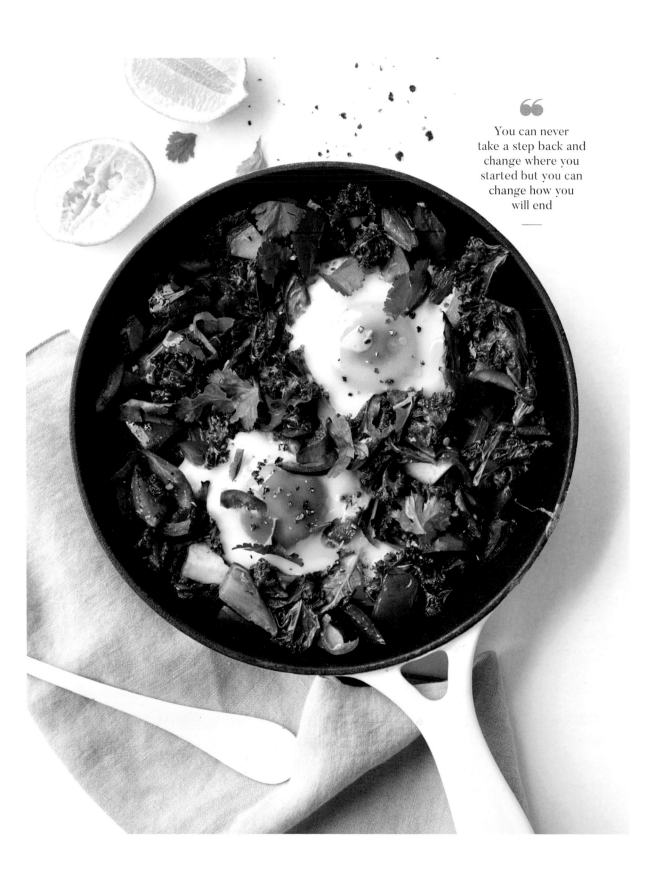

> You can never
> take a step back and
> change where you
> started but you can
> change how you
> will end

breakfast toast

239 CALORIES / 20G CARBS / 15G FAT / 8G PROTEIN

Who doesn't love sweet and nutty flavours? This is a great recipe for that perfect earthy crunch in the morning. I sometimes replace the cinnamon with pumpkin spice to give this dish a more autumnal flavour.

Pop your bread in the toaster. When ready, spread with your favourite nut butter and sprinkle with a handful of blueberries, pumpkin seeds and coconut flakes. Sprinkle with ground cinnamon and drizzle maple syrup over the top.

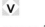

serves 1

1 slice of wholegrain toast
 (gluten-free, if needed)
1–2 tablespoons nut butter
 (almond butter is my fave)
a small handful of blueberries
1 teaspoon pumpkin seeds (omega
 seed mix, if you have it)
1 teaspoon coconut flakes
¼ teaspoon ground cinnamon
½ teaspoon maple syrup

overnight oats

142 CALORIES / 22G CARBS / 4G FAT / 4G PROTEIN

A simple option for those who would much rather stay in bed for those extra 10 minutes... Words can't express how much I love overnight oats. Words also can't express how much I love sleeping. It's a Madden-family favourite – both overnight oats and hitting the snooze button! The oats are extra creamy, extra delicious and super filling.

Add the ingredients to a food storage container in the order listed. Do not stir. Refrigerate overnight.

In the morning, stir the mixture and add a topping of choice, such as blueberries, raspberries, seeds or nut butter. You can also add flavoured protein powder with the almond milk. Eat at home or enjoy on the go.

serves 1

30g gluten-free rolled oats
½ teaspoon vanilla extract
120ml water
60ml almond milk

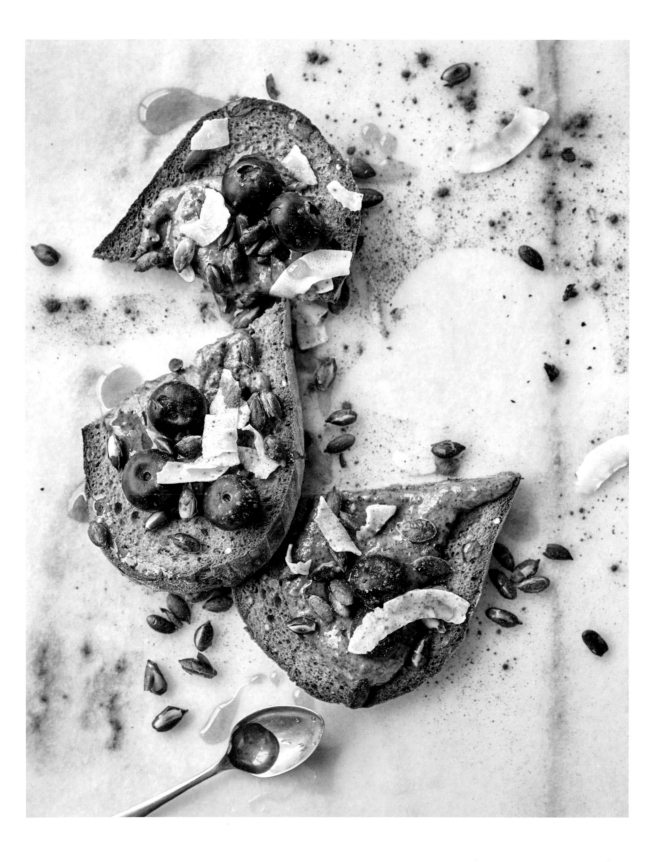

bear bowl

381 CALORIES / 33G CARBS / 17G FAT / 22G PROTEIN

The bear bowl is one of my weekend favourites, especially on a Sunday morning when I have a little more time to enjoy making my breakfast. I call it the bear bowl because it's comforting and packed full of delicious healing ingredients – perfect for lazy, snuggly mornings.

serves 1

2 eggs
½ sweet potato
30g spinach
100g cooked quinoa
1 teaspoon mixed seeds, such as
    sunflower and pumpkin seeds
drizzle of olive oil
salt and freshly ground black
    pepper, to taste

Bring a pan of water to the boil, gently lower in the eggs and cook for 7 minutes. Once cooked, transfer the boiled eggs (aka hot rocks) to a bowl of cold water and peel off the shells.

Cut a criss-cross in the sweet potato and pop it in the microwave for 5–7 minutes on high.

Steam the spinach in a steamer set over a pan of boiling water with the lid on until wilted for 2 minutes.

Combine the sweet potato, spinach and quinoa in a large bowl and toss everything together.

Spoon the sweet potato and quinoa mixture into a bowl and top with the boiled eggs, mixed seeds and drizzle of oil. Season with salt and black pepper.

tip This dish also works well with poached eggs instead of soft-boiled.

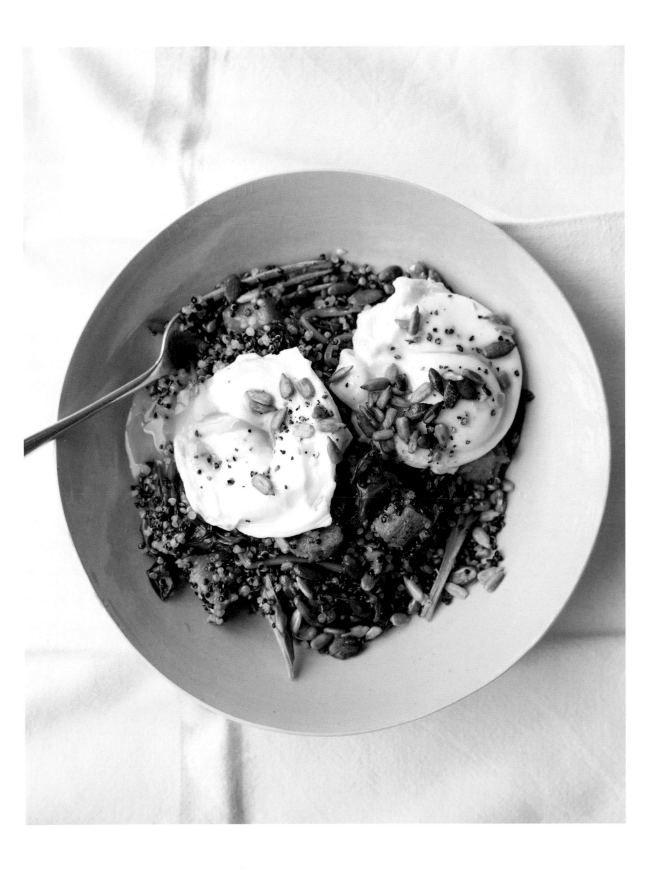

raspberry ripple

270 CALORIES / 33G CARBS / 6G FAT / 21G PROTEIN

Oats are packed with vitamin B, zinc and magnesium. They are a super boost to a gluten-free diet, hence my love for making them a breakfast special.

serves 1

30g gluten-free rolled oats
120ml egg whites
120ml nut milk, such as almond
70g raspberries
1 kiwi, sliced
4 almonds

Mix the oats, egg whites, nut milk and 60ml cold water together in a small saucepan and cook the oats according to packet instructions.

Transfer the oats to a serving bowl and top with the raspberries, kiwi and almonds.

clean crunchy nut

300 CALORIES / 35G CARBS / 8.5G FAT / 21.4G PROTEIN

Struggling to ditch the high-sugar breakfast cereal? Look no further for the solution. I've created this delicious combination of crunchy nut, high-protein, healthy sweetness, which is packed full of nutrients to keep you fuller for longer.

serves 1

30g gluten-free rolled oats
½ banana
60ml nut milk, such as almond
¼ teaspoon ground cinnamon
¼ teaspoon grated nutmeg
¼ teaspoon ground ginger
1 teaspoon nut butter
4 almonds
1 teaspoon maple syrup
120ml beaten egg or egg whites
   (optional, see Tip)

Put the oats, banana, nut milk and 60ml cold water into a small saucepan and cook over a medium heat for 3–4 minutes until the mixture is the consistency you like. Stir in the cinnamon, nutmeg, ginger and nut butter.

Spoon into a serving bowl and top with almonds or mixed nuts and the maple syrup.

tip If you are looking for some extra protein (which I always am!), you can mix some egg or egg white into the oats. Stir fast! A quick beat of a fork is best, and you can't taste the egg at all! Winning.

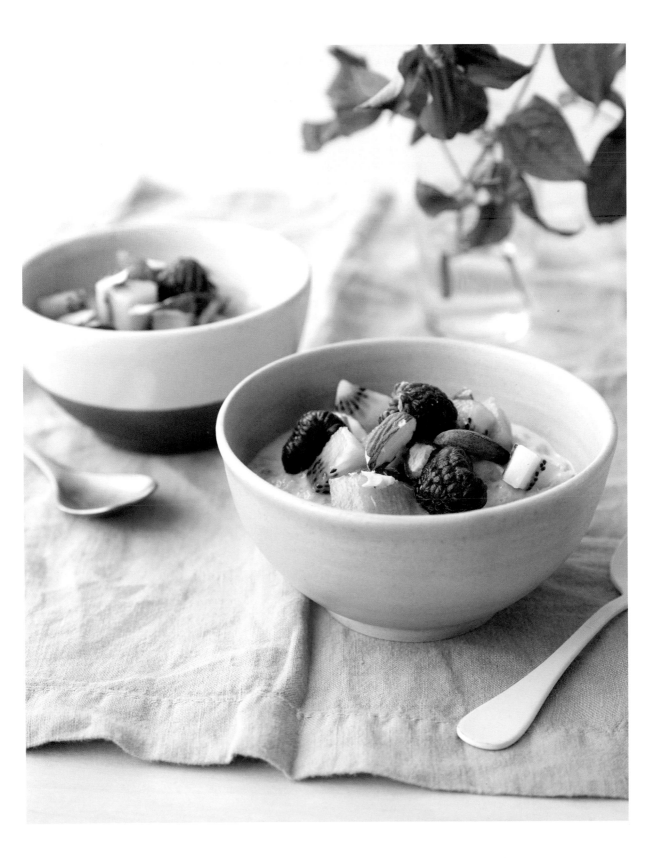

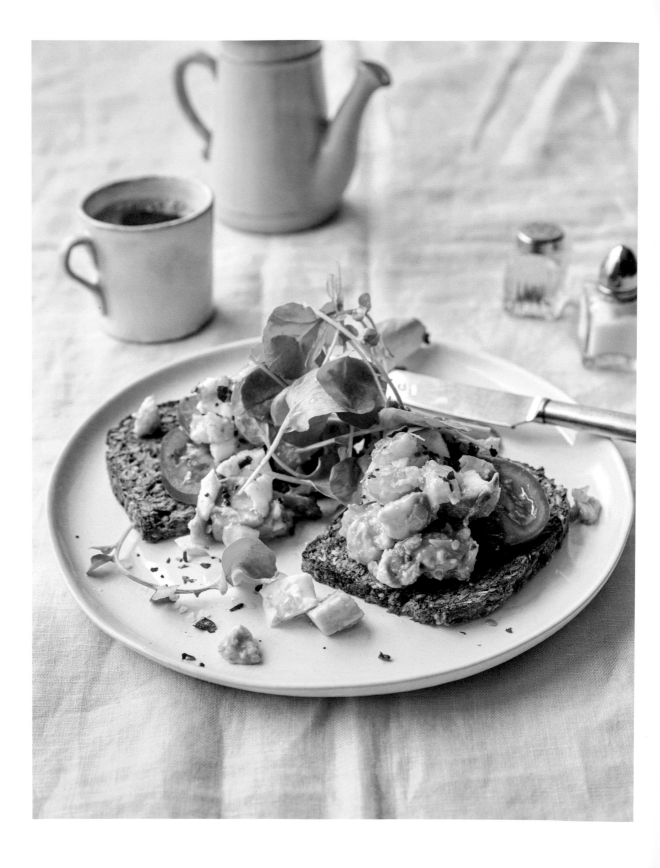

eggocado toast

372 CALORIES / 17G CARBS / 26G FAT / 19G PROTEIN

Eggs are good, avocado is awesome – mix them together and put it on toast and life just got a whole lot better. Yes, it is the Insta symbol of trendy brunches, so make my delicious recipe at home and indulge in its eggocado awesomeness with friends.

Pop the bread in the toaster.

Scoop out the avocado flesh and mash in a bowl with one of the cooked eggs and just the white from the other cooked egg.

Top the toast with a handful of rocket and the chunky eggocado mash. Sprinkle with chilli flakes and finish with a squeeze of lime.

serves 1

2 slices of gluten-free
    multiseed bread
½ avocado, halved and stoned
2 boiled eggs
a handful of rocket
¼ teaspoon chilli flakes
1 lime wedge, to serve

berry beauty bliss

235 CALORIES / 29G CARBS / 4G FAT / 20G PROTEIN

As far as health and beauty benefits go, this is beauty in a bowl. We all know that berries are delicious and we are told that they are good for us, but do you know exactly what their amazing benefits are? Berries are among the richest antioxidant foods on Earth; they are packed with vitamin C – at a much higher level than in oranges – and are known to hydrate the skin and increase skin collagen. So eat up and enjoy your edible face mask.

serves 1

30g gluten-free rolled oats
120ml egg whites
120ml nut milk, plus extra to serve
2 strawberries, hulled and sliced
75g blueberries

Mix the oats, egg whites, nut milk and 60ml cold water together in a small saucepan and cook the oats according to packet instructions.

Spoon into a serving bowl and top with the strawberries and the blueberries. Pour over a little extra nut milk and enjoy.

peanut butter banana oats

178 CALORIES / 22G CARBS / 6G FAT / 11G PROTEIN

PB&B – three little letters I love to see come together. I've never quite been the fan of PB&J, thus I have created the PB&B breakfast special.

Since the original peanut butter and jelly combo is made with white toasted bread and jam, it is not the healthiest start to your day. We want to eat good to feel good, so go ahead, give it a try. This will make you smile even more on the frostiest of mornings.

serves 2

30g gluten-free rolled oats
1 banana, sliced (save a few slices
 to serve)
½ teaspoon chia seeds, plus extra
 to serve
1 teaspoon ground cinnamon
a pinch of sea salt
240ml water, nut milk or a blend
of both,
 plus extra to serve
1 tablespoon peanut butter or any
 nut butter
maple syrup, to serve (optional)
120ml beaten egg or egg whites
 (optional, see Tip, page 28)

Put the oats, banana, chia seeds, cinnamon and sea salt in a pan over a medium-high heat. Add the water or milk and stir to combine. Cook for 3-4 minutes, or until all the liquid has been absorbed. Stir the oats several times while cooking to make sure the banana slices melt into the oats and the chia seeds don't clump together. You'll know the oatmeal is done when all the liquid is absorbed and the oats are thick and fluffy.

Divide the oats between two bowls and serve with the peanut butter, reserved banana slices and a sprinkle of chia seeds. Add a splash of milk and/or maple syrup on top before serving, if desired.

tip Add a few frozen raspberries if you really do love PB&J.

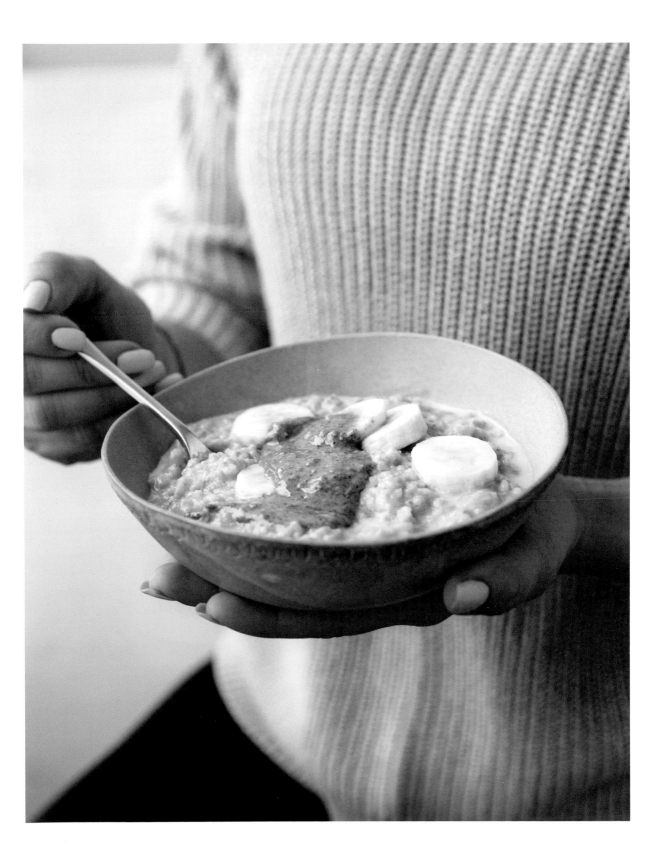

good morning miami

227 CALORIES / 4G CARBS / 17G FAT / 16G PROTEIN

It was during an extended stay in Miami that I woke up to enjoy this bloat-free, protein-packed, light but ever-so-satisfying breakfast before hitting the beach. It is certainly a summer slimming saviour.

serves 1

½ teaspoon coconut oil

6 plum tomatoes, halved

½ avocado, halved, stoned, peeled and sliced

120ml egg whites

30g spinach

1 tablespoon chopped coriander

salt and freshly ground black pepper, to taste

Preheat the grill. Lightly grease an ovenproof frying pan with the coconut oil and set over a low heat. Add the tomatoes and avocado to the pan. Meanwhile, whisk the egg whites and 60ml cold water together in a bowl. Add the spinach and coriander. Pour the mixture into the frying pan over the tomatoes and avocado. Cook for 3–4 minutes until the omelette is nearly set, then pop under the grill to cook the top until cooked to the desired consistency. Season with salt and pepper.

supremo breakfast smoothie

247 CALORIES / 24G CARBS / 11G FAT / 11G PROTEIN

My good morning Supremo. I have a real soft spot for this delicious smoothie; it's got everything I need, and more often than not I will blitz this up every morning. You need not miss breakfast if you have these ingredients to hand, as it's a super-quick and easy recipe that can be made in less than 2 minutes. It's bouncing full of energy-boosting nutrients, so you can easily skip coffee, too. Stay smiling with Supremo.

serves 2

4 strawberries

100g blueberries

100g raspberries

30g spinach

2 teaspoons chia seeds

2 teaspoons flaxseeds

1 teaspoon maca powder

1 teaspoon camu camu powder

1 tablespoon nut butter, such as almond

20g protein powder

25g gluten-free rolled oats

Add all the ingredients to a blender, reserving some of the chia seeds and fruit, and blitz until smooth. Top with the reserved chia seeds and fruit.

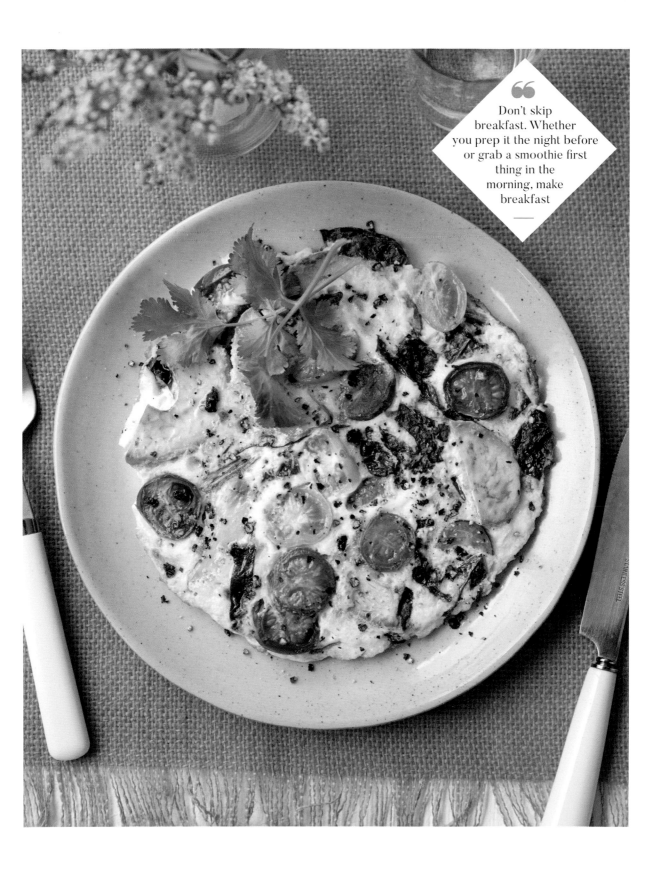

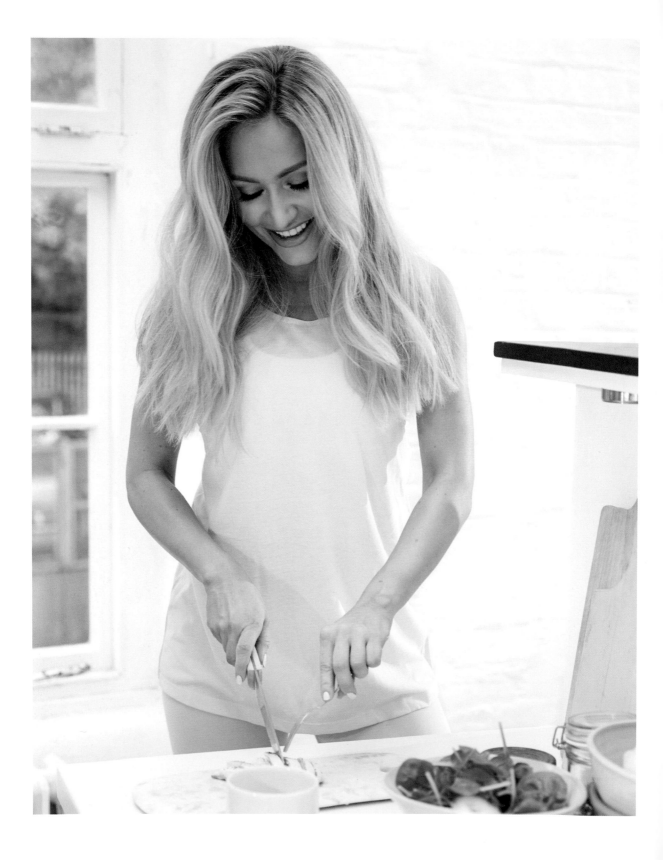

light meals

chicks in a boat

87 CALORIES / 5G CARBS / 7G FAT / 3G PROTEIN PER BOAT

This recipe has it all: so many flavours, so many textures, a truly great recipe to introduce your strictly carnivore friends to veganism.

V

serves 3

400g can chickpeas, drained and
   rinsed
1 teaspoon ground turmeric
1 teaspoon chilli powder
1 spring onion (green part only),
   chopped
1 garlic clove, chopped (optional)
6 mint leaves
1 teaspoon ground cumin
1 tablespoon sesame seeds
1 tablespoon flaxseeds
1 tablespoon olive oil
6 large lettuce leaves, to serve

FOR THE AVOCADO MIX
2 avocados, halved, stoned and
   roughly chopped
2 tomatoes, chopped
1 tablespoon lime juice
1 spring onion (green part only),
   finely sliced
a bunch of basil leaves, torn
1 green pepper, deseeded and
   finely chopped
6 crushed walnuts
salt, to taste

First make the avocado mix. In a medium mixing bowl, smash up the avocados and tomatoes. Add the lime juice and mix until smooth. You can pop it into a blender if you prefer, but I like it chunky. Mix in the remaining ingredients, but only half the crushed walnuts, and season with a little salt.

Put the chickpeas, turmeric and chilli powder in a pan over a medium heat. Pour in 60ml water and cook for 3 minutes. Once all the water has been absorbed, add the remaining ingredients, except the lettuce, and stir for roughly 1 minute. Remove the pan from the heat and cover with a lid.

Wash and dry the lettuce leaves – these will be used as your boats. Fill the lettuce boats with 2 tablespoons of avocado mix and 2 tablespoons of chickpeas. Sprinkle with the reserved walnuts. Serve and enjoy.

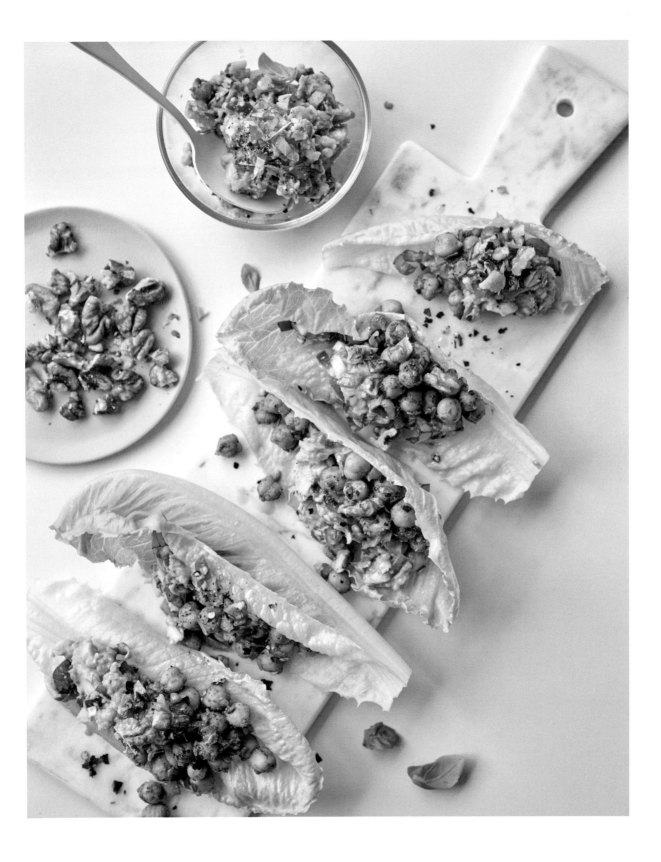

power bowl

599 CALORIES / 35.5G CARBS / 34G FAT / 38.5G PROTEIN (WITH DRESSING)

Have you just hit the gym really hard, and are now feeling full of happy endorphins but slightly exhausted? This power bowl will revitalise you completely, packed with good carbs, protein and fats, it's a bowl of balance.

serves 1

100g sweet potato, peeled and
   cubed
¼ teaspoon coconut oil, melted,
   plus extra for the chicken
1 skinless chicken breast fillet
30g spinach, chopped
4 walnut halves, chopped
25g blueberries or raspberries
50g cooked quinoa

**FOR THE CREAMY
AVOCADO DRESSING**
¼ ripe avocado, halved, stoned
   and chopped
30g coriander
2 tablespoons lime juice
½ teaspoon salt

Preheat the oven to 180°C/gas mark 4.

Mix the sweet potato with the coconut oil to coat and evenly spread the cubes over a baking sheet. Roast for 25 minutes. Pop the chicken in a baking dish, rub a little coconut oil over it and place in the oven at the same time as the sweet potato.

Add the spinach, walnuts, berries and quinoa to a large mixing bowl. Shred the cooked chicken with a knife and add both the chicken and sweet potato to the mixing bowl. Toss everything together.

To make the dressing, put all the ingredients in a blender and blitz until smooth. Coat the chicken mix with 1 tablespoon of dressing and enjoy.

tip   The leftover dressing can be used for any other salad. It will keep in the fridge for up to 3 days.

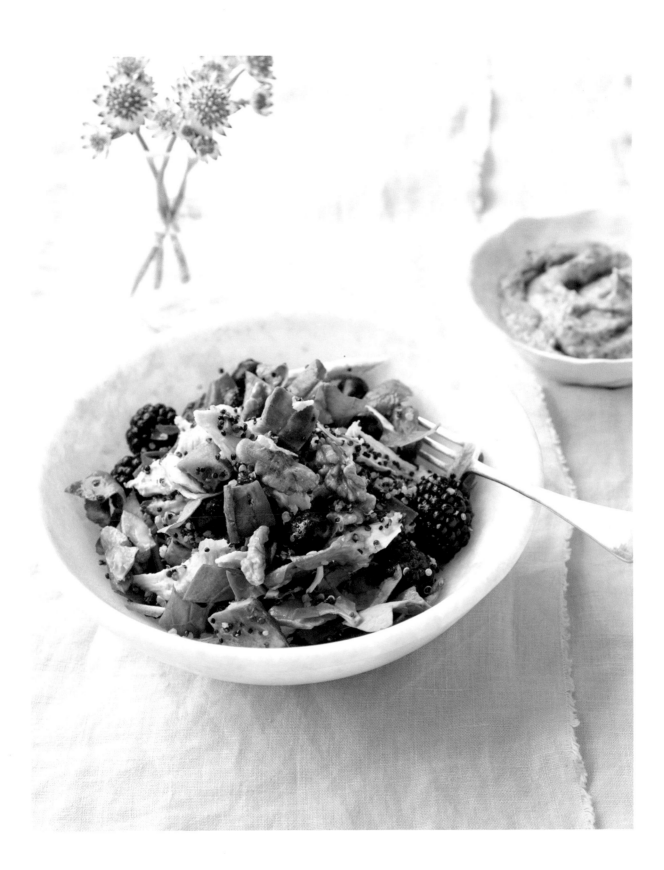

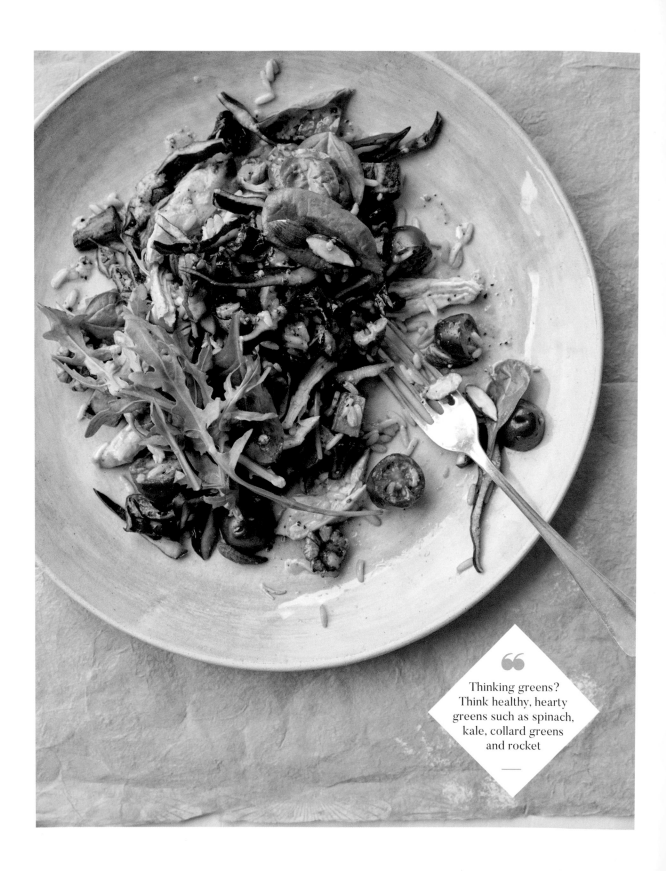

> Thinking greens?
> Think healthy, hearty
> greens such as spinach,
> kale, collard greens
> and rocket

winter harvest salad

824 CALORIES / 65G CARBS / 47G FAT / 45G PROTEIN (WITH DRESSING)

Nourish your body with this welcoming winter salad. Cooking by season is the best way to make sure you get the most flavour out of ingredients, so when winter comes round, be sure to fill up on this hungry harvest bowl.

Preheat the oven to 200°C/gas mark 6. Mix the the sweet potato with the coconut oil and evenly spread the cubes over a baking sheet. Roast for 25 minutes. Pop the chicken in a baking dish, rub a little coconut oil over it and place in the oven at the same time as the sweet potato.

Cook the brown rice according to the packet instructions.

To make the dressing, whisk the mustards, honey and white wine vinegar together in a small bowl or jar. Slowly add the olive oil and build up until you get the consistency you want. To assemble your salad, mix all the ingredinets together in a large bowl then add the dressing to taste.

serves 1

½ sweet potato, peeled and cubed
½ teaspoon coconut oil
1 skinless chicken breast fillet
50g brown rice
15g spinach
15g rocket
1 tablespoon cranberries
5 walnuts, chopped
4 almonds, chopped
8 plum tomatoes, halved
75g red cabbage
1 tablespoon Dijon dressing

FOR THE DRESSING
25ml Dijon mustard
25ml wholegrain mustard
25ml honey
100ml white wine vinegar
400ml extra virgin olive oil

tropical storm

391 CALORIES / 12G CARBS / 25G FAT / 32G PROTEIN

Shout out to my most popular salad, a combination of fruity flavours and tasty textures that make it possibly the best chicken salad ever.

Heat a pan over a medium heat and add the coconut oil. Once the oil has melted, add the chicken and bring to a medium heat.

Meanwhile, put the spinach in a mixing bowl and toss in the chopped fruit and vegetables. Drizzle the olive oil over the salad and mix it all up. When the chicken is cooked, I like to shred it and then scatter it over the bowl.

serves 1

½ teaspoon coconut oil
1 skinless chicken breast fillet, diced
30g spinach
8 plum tomatoes, chopped into bite-sized chunks
½ avocado, halved, stoned and chopped into bite-sized pieces
75g pineapple, chopped into bite-sized pieces
1 teaspoon extra virgin olive oil

mum's chicken soup

180 CALORIES / 15G CARBS / 7G FAT / 17G PROTEIN

An old Madden household special. Mum created this healthy, comforting recipe for cold afternoons when we got home from school or dance practice, and it's no surprise why. This recipe is perfect for when the seasons change and the days get shorter. Getting in from work or the gym and tucking into this is a great way to get your nutrients, relax and stay warm.

serves 4

1 teaspoon coconut oil

2 leeks, chopped into chunks

4 carrots, chopped into chunks

6 celery sticks, chopped into chunks

1 litre boiling water

2 vegetable stock cubes

1 sweet potato, diced into cubes

230g chicken thighs, roughly chopped

a bunch of flat-leaf parsley, finely chopped

Pop a large saucepan over a medium heat. Add the coconut oil and melt, then throw in the leeks, carrots and celery and stir to coat in the oil.

Crumble the stock cubes into a jug and pour in the boiling water, stirring to dissolve.

Add the sweet potato to the pan, then pour over the stock, add the chicken and bring to the boil. Simmer for a good 30 minutes, stirring often. Add the parsley and simmer for a further 15–20 minutes. Serve and enjoy.

tip This soup can be blitzed in a blender, that's how my mummy does it!

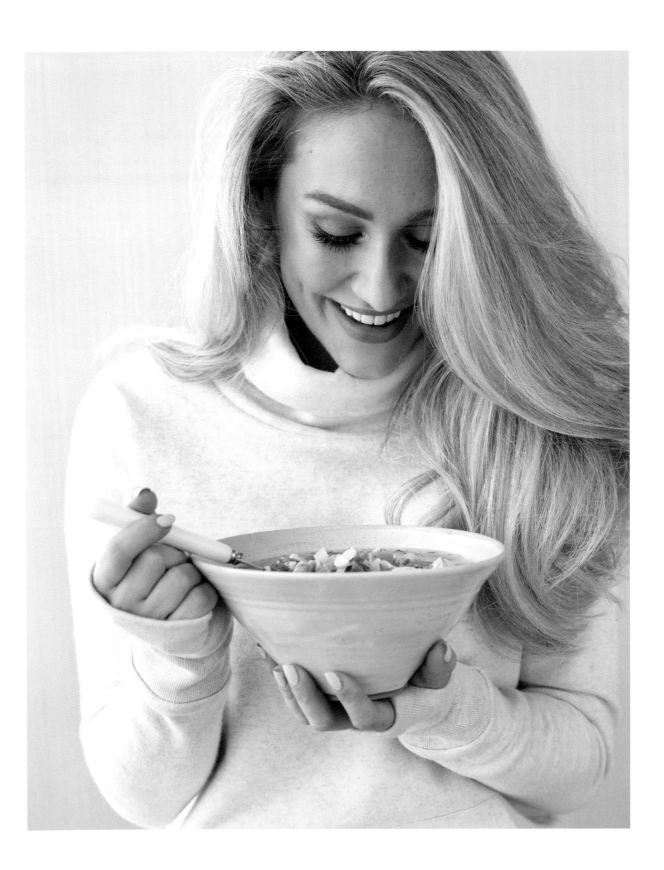

prawn star

163 CALORIES / 6G CARBS / 7G FAT / 20G PROTEIN

Looking for something fresh, light and delicious? Look no further. Who doesn't love the taste of zesty prawns? Combining fresh flavours with a good protein source is the perfect recipe for energy and vitality.

serves 1

60g lettuce, finely shredded
75g red cabbage, finely shredded
¼ red pepper, deseeded and
    finely diced
4 mint leaves, thinly sliced
15g coriander leaves, thinly sliced
100g cooked king prawns
salt and freshly ground black
    pepper, to taste

FOR THE DRESSING
1 teaspoon extra virgin olive oil
squeeze of lime juice
1 teaspoon sesame seeds

Combine the lettuce and cabbage in a large salad bowl. Add the red pepper, mint and coriander leaves, and toss to mix.

To make the dressing, mix the oil, lime juice and sesame seeds together in a
small bowl.

Top the salad with the prawns, drizzle over the dressing and season to taste.

tunacado

serves 2

1 medium avocado, halved and
    stoned
120g can tuna in spring water,
    drained
½ red pepper, deseeded and
    roughly chopped
½ jalapeño pepper (optional)
a bunch of coriander (15g), finely
    chopped
squeeze of lime

215 CALORIES / 3.4G CARBS / 15G FAT / 17G PROTEIN

Pretty much the tornado of my recipes. This is super quick to prep, super easy to make and super tasty. If you're looking to make a meal in whirlwind speed, this is the one for you. Smash everything in a bowl and munch up.

Scoop out some of the flesh from the avocado halves to widen the 'bowl' area. Place the scooped-out avocado into a mixing bowl and mash with a fork. Add the tuna, red pepper, jalapeño (if using) and coriander. Squeeze the lime juice over the top. Mix until everything is mushy.

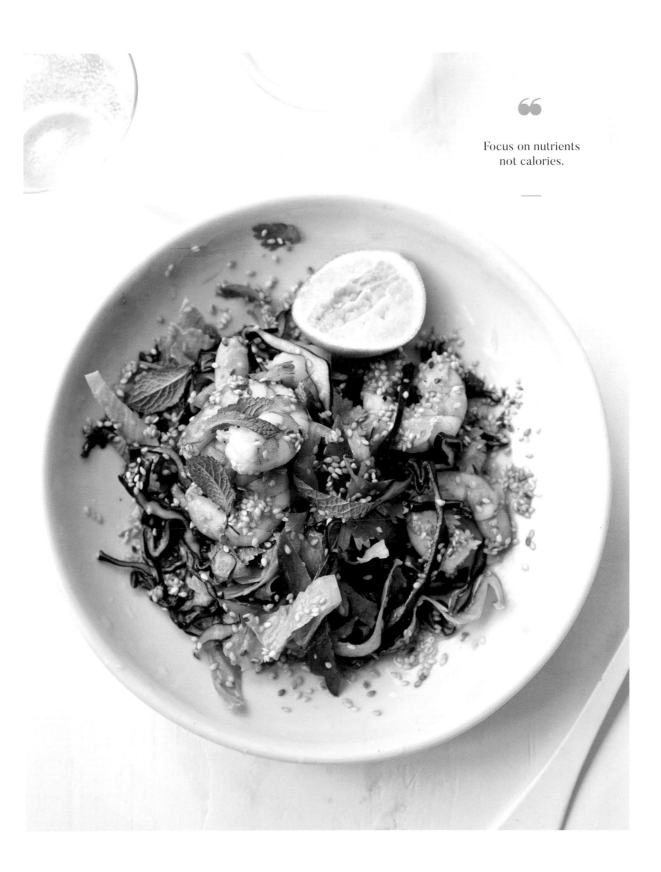

66

Focus on nutrients
not calories.

—

beauty bite

335 CALORIES / 28G CARBS / 20G FAT / 11G PROTEIN

The name says it all. What a beautifully flavoured recipe, so fresh. I have this in the morning, or sometimes if I'm craving something sweet in the evening this is the perfect choice.

serves 1

180g coconut yogurt

1 teaspoon maple syrup or honey

75g berries, such as blueberries, raspberries or blackberries (I use frozen)

6 walnut halves, chopped

1 teaspoon pumpkin seeds

1 teaspoon nut butter, such as almond (optional)

In a bowl, mix the yogurt with the maple syrup. Top with the berries, walnuts and pumpkin seeds, and if you like, a little nut butter.

tofu toast

338 CALORIES / 17G CARBS / 25G FAT / 13G PROTEIN

This is a great vegan recipe for the day after you've exercised. All your protein has been used up overnight to repair your body, so this will kickstart that toning muscle growth.

V

serves 2

1 tablespoon coconut oil

10 cherry tomatoes, halved

1 spring onion (green part only), sliced

½ red chilli, sliced

200g tofu

½ teaspoon ground turmeric

2 slices of bread (gluten-free if you wish)

1 avocado, halved, stoned and sliced

salt and freshly ground black pepper, to taste

Heat half the oil in a frying pan over a low–medium heat. Place the tomatoes in the pan, cut-side down, and fry until soft. Remove from the pan and set aside.

Heat the remaining coconut oil over a medium heat and add the spring onion and chilli. Add the tofu and break it up with a fork into chunks. Sprinkle over the turmeric and a little salt and stir in the pan. Your tofu should be looking quite like scrambled eggs now.

Pop the bread in the toaster and return the tomatoes to the pan, stirring to heat through. Smash the avocado and spread it onto the toast. Add a little tofu mountain on top and season. Enjoy this delicious vegan yumminess any time of day.

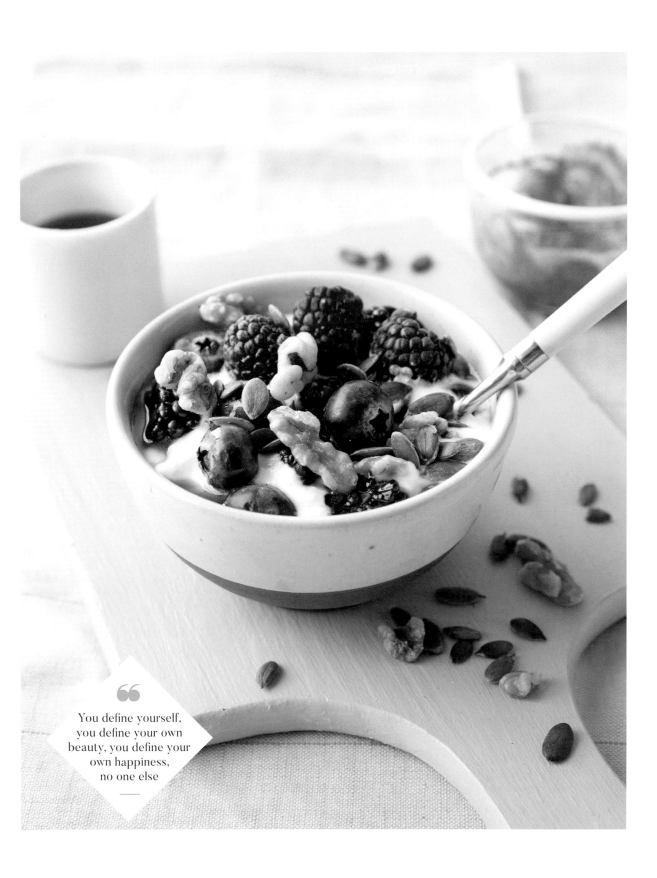

cheat-free cheese rolls

180 CALORIES / 3.7G CARBS / 10.2G FAT / 18.6G PROTEIN

Let's be real here, who doesn't love cheese? I find it is often difficult to eat cheese and get away with it, especially when trying to tackle the bloat. Do not fear, 1 tablespoon of feta shouldn't do too much bloating damage so these cheese rolls are perfect for feeding your cheese obsession.

serves 1

1 egg, plus 2 egg whites

60ml water

¼ teaspoon coconut oil

30g spinach

4 plum tomatoes, chopped into small pieces

1 tablespoon of feta, crumbled, plus extra to garnish (optional)

15g rocket

Beat the egg, egg whites and water in a small bowl until blended.

Heat the oil in a non-stick pan over a medium heat. Gently pour in the egg mixture so it covers the entire pan. When the egg is beginning to set a little, place your filling of spinach, tomatoes and feta on one side of the pan. When the egg is almost fully set, use a spatula to gently roll the egg over, starting on the filling side. Continue to cook your egg roll for a few more seconds until completely set.

Gently place the roll on a plate and sprinkle a little feta on top, if you wish. Garnish with a side of rocket and enjoy.

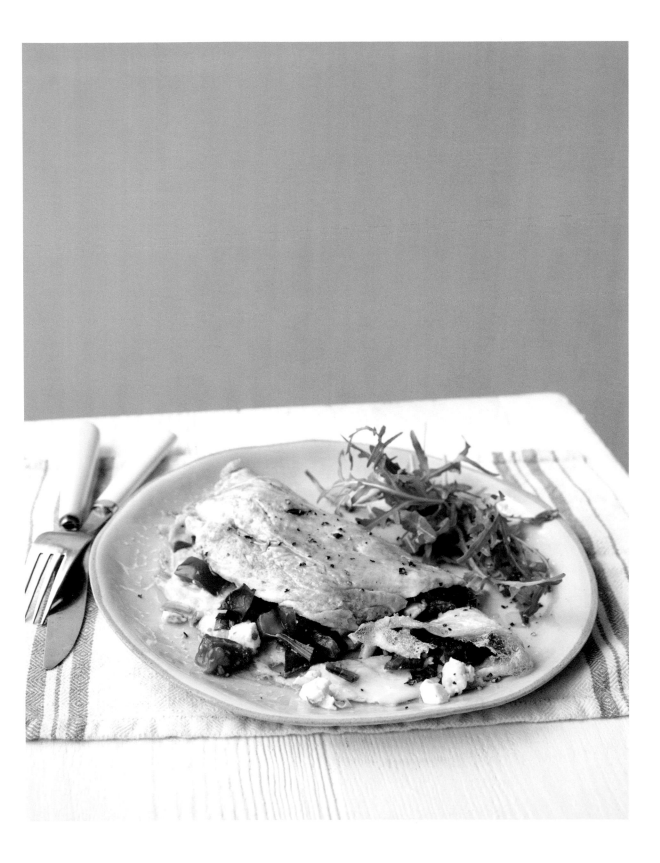

taste the rainbow

584 CALORIES / 31G CARBS / 32G FAT / 44G PROTEIN (WITHOUT DRESSING)

This is not only the prettiest of salads but it is bursting with flavour as well as nutrients. Start eating for the body you want, not the body you have. Nobody is built like you, you design yourself.

serves 2

½ tablespoon coconut oil
2 skinless chicken breast fillets, diced
1 teaspoon chilli powder
120g blueberries
100g lettuce, chopped
70g chopped almonds
100g sun-dried tomatoes
2 teaspoons extra virgin olive oil
salt and freshly ground black pepper, to taste

FOR THE DRESSING
25g Dijon mustard
25g wholegrain mustard
25g clear honey
100ml white wine vinegar
400ml extra virgin olive oil

Heat the coconut oil in a large pan over a medium heat. Sprinkle the chicken with the chilli powder, salt and black pepper. Add the chicken to the pan and cook through until you get a gorgeous golden colour on all sides.

When the chicken is fully cooked, set aside to cool and prep all the fruits and veggies. I like to chop everything up and toss it into a big salad bowl.

To make the dressing, whisk the mustards, honey and vinegar together in a small bowl or jar. Slowly add the olive oil, whisking or shaking between each addition, until you get the consistency you want.

When the chicken is cool, add it to the salad bowl and drizzle over the dressing. Serve and enjoy.

tip The dressing recipe makes enough for 8 servings and can be stored in a jar in the fridge for up to 10 days.

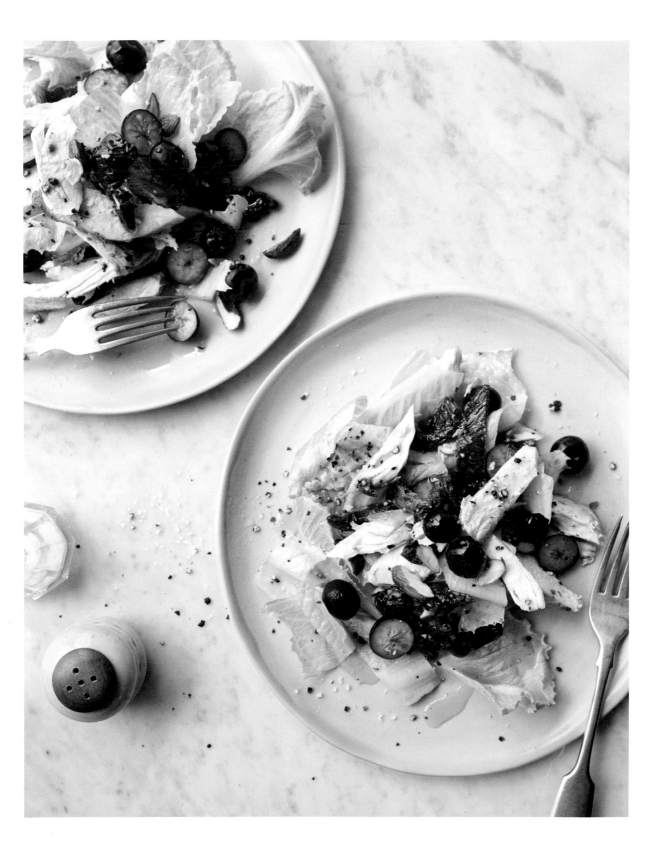

chunky avocado toast

398 CALORIES / 19G CARBS / 28G FAT / 18G PROTEIN

Another weekend morning classic. Avocado toast has become a breakfast staple, and for good reason – it's quick, simple and hugely healthy. Nothing feels better than waking up on a relaxing, carefree weekend and indulging in hot toast topped with soft, squishy avocado and oozing eggs.

serves 1

2 eggs
½ avocado, halved and stoned
juice of ½ lime
a pinch of chilli flakes
a pinch each of flaky salt and
    freshly ground black pepper
1 slice of gluten-free bread
¼ teaspoon olive oil

Fill a large saucepan with water and bring to the boil. Add the eggs and boil for 5–7 minutes, depending on how gooey you would like them to be.

Scoop out the avocado and in a small bowl, roughly mash it, then add the lime juice and chilli flakes and season well with black pepper.

Toast the bread and drizzle over the olive oil.

Remove the eggs from the pan and rinse well under cold water. Carefully remove the shells when cool enough to handle.

Top the toasted bread with the chunky avocado and then the boiled eggs and season with a little salt.

tip Flaky salt is key for adding that extra crunch.

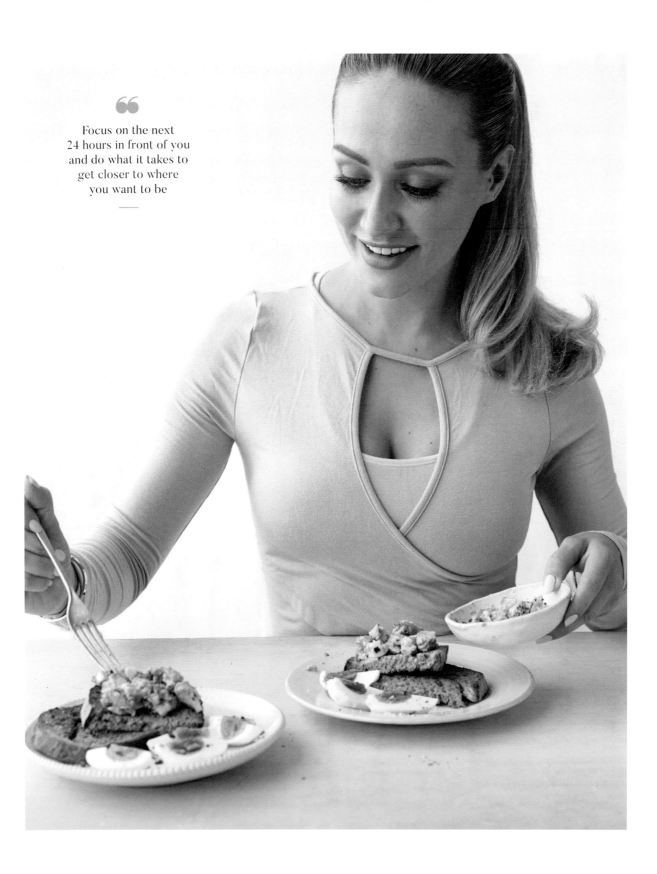

snappy happy

355 CALORIES / 45G CARBS / 16G FAT / 12G PROTEIN

This is one of my easiest meals; it's perfect to prep beforehand so all you need to do is pop it in the oven and wait. So simple. So wholesome. I always peel cucumber as I find the skin leaves me a little burpy. I like to remove the skins from the chickpeas, too, but this can be time consuming.

serves 1

1 small sweet potato, cut into
    wedges
¼ teaspoon ground cinnamon
1 tablespoon olive oil
½ x 400g can chickpeas, drained
    and rinsed
½ teaspoon chilli flakes
a handful of rocket or spinach
⅓ large cucumber, peeled and
sliced
6 cherry tomatoes, halved
½ teaspoon maple syrup
1 tablespoon lemon juice
salt, to taste

Preheat the oven to 180°C/gas mark 4.

Mix the sweet potato, cinnamon, olive oil and a sprinkle of salt together in a mixing bowl. Transfer to a roasting dish and roast in the oven for 30 minutes. I like my sweet potatoes soft and squishy.

Pop the chickpeas on top of the sweet potato, sprinkle with chilli flakes and return to the oven for a further 30 minutes.

Mix the rocket or spinach, cucumber and tomatoes together with the maple syrup and lemon juice. Stir in the sweet potato and chickpeas.

Transfer to a bowl and serve.

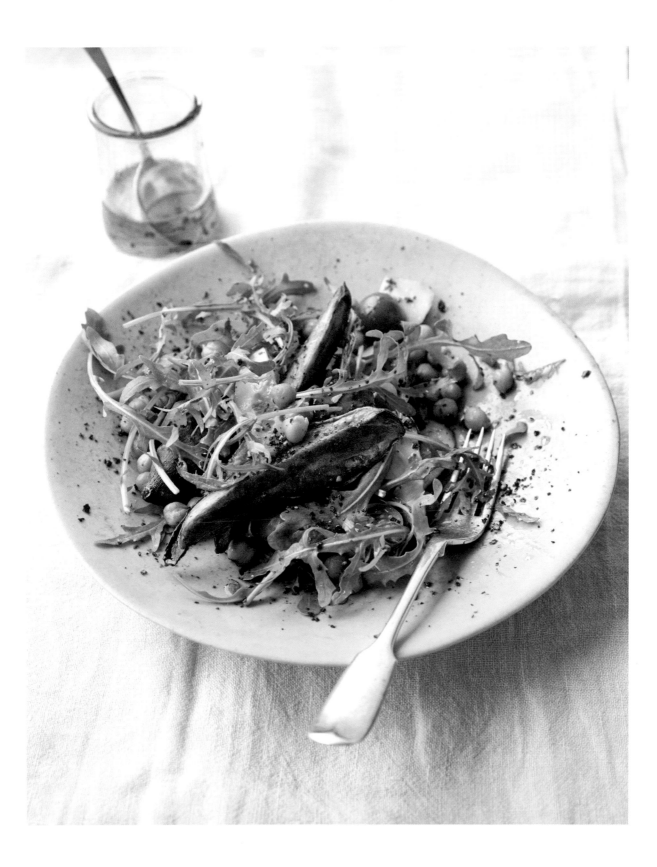

chicken à la queen

298 CALORIES / 0.1G CARBS / 12G FAT / 47G PROTEIN

When we are eating for strong not skinny, I suggest you indulge in this recipe for post-workout protein power.

serves 1

1 skinless chicken breast fillet
½ teaspoon coconut oil
1 egg, plus 3 egg whites
30g spinach
salt and freshly ground black
    pepper, to taste

Preheat the grill to high. Grill the chicken breast for 5 minutes on each side.

Heat a pan with the coconut oil over a low heat.

Whisk the egg and egg whites together, add the spinach to the mix, pour into the pan and scramble over a low heat, stirring continuously.

Cut the cooked chicken into cubes and mix with the scrambled eggs. Season and serve.

curry avocado chicken boats

449 CALORIES / 10G CARBS / 29G FAT / 37G PROTEIN

Here is a fun recipe for the whole family. If you are like me, you love foods that are super creamy and super delicious. Takeaway cravings can be changed up with this simple recipe. The smoothness of the sauce along with the crunch of the lettuce and almonds make for the perfect tasty combo.

serves 2

½ tablespoon vegan mayonnaise
1 tablespoon coconut yogurt
1 teaspoon curry powder
a pinch of ground cinnamon
1½ avocados, halved, stoned and
    roughly sliced
2 skinless chicken breast fillets,
    grilled and shredded
3 dried or fresh apricots, diced
5-6 Little Gem lettuce leaves
1 tablespoon flaked or crushed
    almonds
salt and freshly ground black
    pepper, to taste

Mix the mayonnaise, yogurt, curry powder and cinnamon together, adding a splash of water if the sauce is too thick.

In a small bowl, mash the avocados into soft but still chunky pieces.

Mix the sauce, avocados, chicken and apricots together. Season with salt and black pepper. Separate out the lettuce leaves and pack the curried chicken and avocado into them. Top with the flaked or crushed almonds.

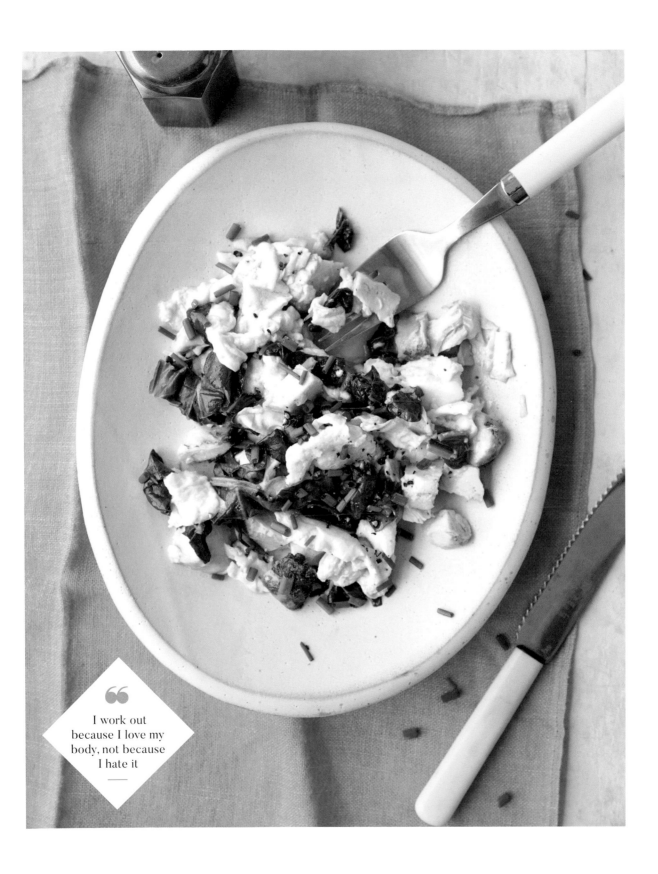

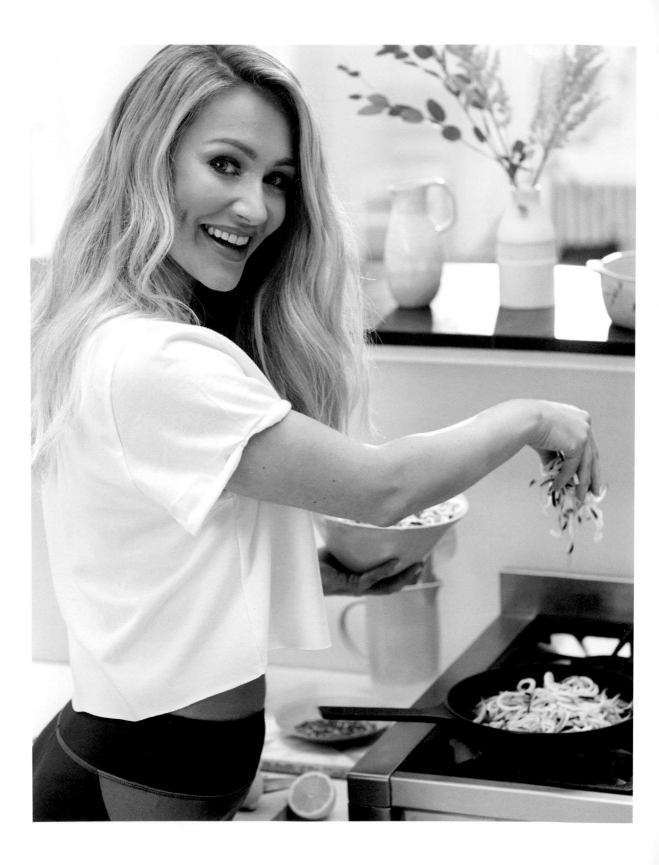

main meals

thai green curry

497 CALORIES / 10G CARBS / 31G FAT / 46G PROTEIN

It's lean, it's mean and it's green! Packed full of aromatic herbs and spices, this curry is an absolute taste sensation! Marry that with lean chicken breasts and cauliflower rice and it's a sure-fire way to keep your diet on track without it becoming stale and lifeless. Takeaway curries will be a thing of the past.

serves 4

600g skinless chicken breast, diced
400ml can coconut milk
120ml chicken stock or water
1 teaspoon fish sauce
1 teaspoon coconut palm sugar or ½ teaspoon stevia
2 red peppers, deseeded and cut into strips
100g baby corn
a small handful of spring onions (green parts only), cut into strips

FOR THE CURRY PASTE
2 lemongrass stalks, thinly sliced
3-4 green chillies, deseeded
4 spring onions (green parts only)
1 tablespoon freshly grated ginger
25g chopped coriander, plus extra to serve
25g Thai basil, plus extra to garnish
1 teaspoon ground coriander
1 teapoon ground cumin
1 teaspoon fish sauce
zest of 1 lemon, plus juice of ½
½ teaspoon freshly ground black pepper
2 tablespoons coconut oil

Start by making the curry paste. Add the lemongrass stalks to a food processor with the remaining curry paste ingredients. Whizz together until you end up with a thick, green paste. You will probably need to stop every now and then to scrape the sides down with a spoon to get all the ingredients to blend properly. If you don't have a food processor you can also use a high-powered blender (such as a NutriBullet) – it may take a little longer.

Add the curry paste to a large saucepan and warm over a low heat for 2-3 minutes. Add the chicken and stir, coating it in the curry paste. Cook for 4-5 minutes over a medium heat. Add the coconut milk, chicken stock, fish sauce and sugar or stevia and bring to the boil for 2 minutes.

Reduce the heat and add the red peppers, baby corn and spring onions. Simmer for at least 15 minutes until the sauce thickens.

Serve over cauliflower rice. Garnish with basil or coriander leaves and add an extra squeeze of lemon juice for more brightness. Enjoy.

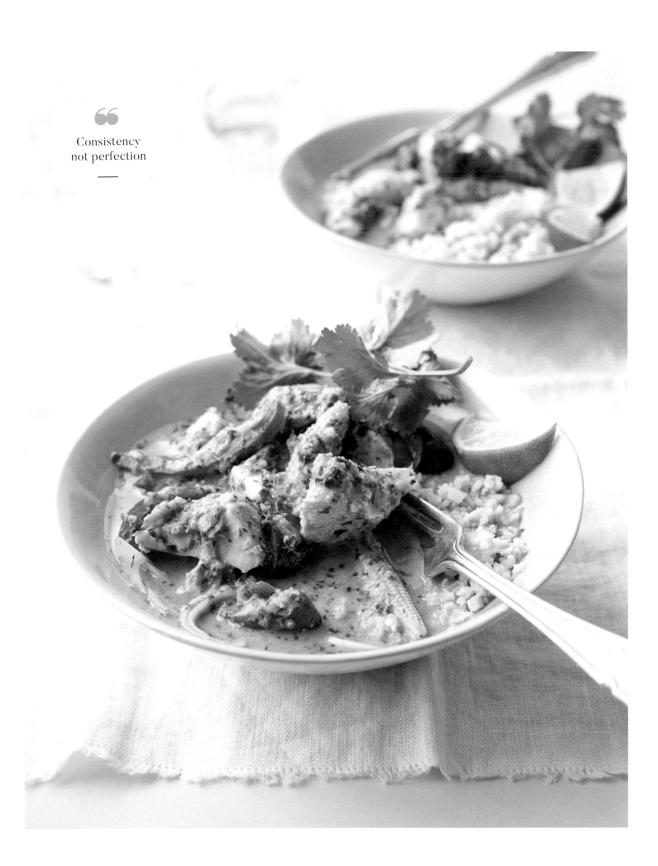

mummy's meatballs

405 CALORIES / 32G CARBS / 15G FAT / 38G PROTEIN (WITH PASTA)

Meatballs! Just like-a mama use to make... well, not quite. With a few sneaky substitutes you can change this Italian classic into a healthy favourite that will help keep you looking like Sophia Loren, not Tony Soprano.

serves 4

FOR THE MEATBALLS
350g lean high-quality beef mince
1 garlic clove, crushed
a pinch of dried chilli flakes
1 dessertspoon tomato purée
a dash of Worcestershire sauce
1 egg, beaten
60g mozzarella
30g Parmesan, grated, plus extra
   to serve
      (optional)

FOR THE TOMATO SAUCE
60g unsmoked back bacon,
   fat removed
1 onion, finely chopped
1 garlic clove, crushed
1 dessertspoon cornflour
250ml vegetable stock
2 tomatoes, chopped
400g can chopped tomatoes
1 tablespoon chopped basil leaves,
   plus extra to serve (optional)
salt and freshly ground black
   pepper, to taste

300g cauliflower rice or
   200g cooked spelt pasta,
   to serve

Thoroughly mix all the meatball ingredients together in a bowl, apart from the mozzarella and Parmesan. Using clean, wet hands, roll the meatballs, incorporating a piece of mozzarella in the centre of each and place them in an ovenproof dish. Cover with clingfilm and set aside in the fridge until the sauce is ready.

Preheat the oven to 180°C/gas mark 4.

To make the sauce, fry the bacon in a saucepan over a medium heat until golden brown. Add the onion and the garlic and cook for 1–2 minutes without browning. Remove from the heat and stir in the cornflour. Add the stock, then the fresh and canned tomatoes and return to the hob. Bring to the boil, stirring all the time, and cook until the sauce thickens. Finally, stir in the basil and remove the pan from the heat.

Take the meatballs out of the fridge and remove the clingfilm, then pour over the sauce and sprinkle with the Parmesan. Cover the dish with foil and bake for 35 minutes. Remove the foil and cook for a further 10 minutes.

Serve with cauliflower rice or spelt pasta and a few basil leaves and sprinkle of grated Parmesan, if you wish.

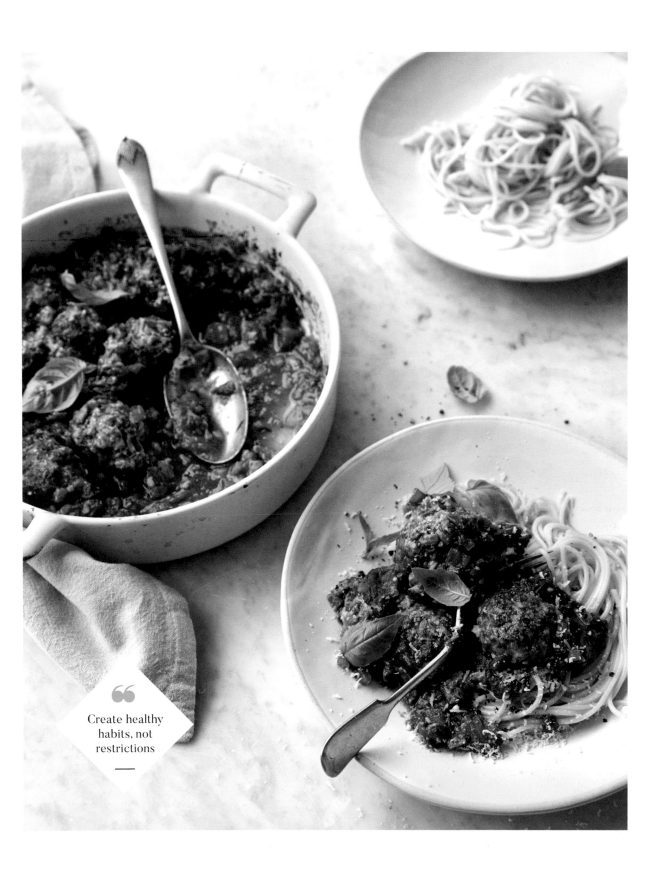

Create healthy
habits, not
restrictions
—

living fajita loca

415 CALORIES / 31G CARBS / 14G FAT / 47G PROTEIN (WITHOUT GUACAMOLE)
120 CALORIES / 8G CARBS / 10G FAT / 1.5G PROTEIN (GUACAMOLE)

If it's date night or Ricky Martin happens to pop over for dinner, you have got to serve my Friday fajita special. Heat some gluten-free tortillas and wrap and roll your own tasty fajitas.

serves 4

3 tablespoons olive oil

juice of ½ lime, plus
   2 tablespoons

1 teaspoon chilli powder

½ teaspoon paprika

½ teaspoon ground cumin

2 garlic cloves, crushed

600g skinless chicken breast
   fillets, cut into strips

1 spring onion (green part only),
   diced

1 red pepper, deseeded and cut
   into strips

1 yellow pepper, deseeded and cut
   into strips

1 green pepper, deseeded and cut
   into strips

15g coriander sprigs

4 gluten-free tortillas, to serve

FOR THE GUACAMOLE

1 tomato

2 avocados

juice of 3 limes

a large handful of finely chopped
   coriander

1 tablespoon Frank's hot sauce
   (optional)

salt and freshly ground black
   pepper, to taste

To make the guacamole, cut the tomato in half and remove the seeds, then finely slice the flesh into tiny cubes. Cut the avocados in half, scoop the flesh into a bowl and mash it up with a fork. Add the remaining ingredients and mix well. Taste for seasoning then scoop into a bowl, ready to serve.

Prepare the rest of the dish. In a bowl, combine 1 tablespoon of the oil with the juice of ½ lime, the chilli powder, paprika, cumin, garlic, salt and black pepper. Add the chicken and toss in the spice mixture to coat.

Preheat 1 tablespoon of the oil in a saucepan over a medium heat, then add half of the chicken and cook for 3–5 minutes until just cooked. Remove from the pan and set aside. Repeat with the remaining chicken.

Add 1 tablespoon of oil to the same pan. Add the spring onion and cook for 2 minutes. Add the peppers and cook for a further 2 minutes or just until hot. Return the chicken to the pan, stir to combine, then add the 2 tablespoons of lime juice.

Garnish with the coriander and serve with a side of guacamole and gluten-free tortillas or iceberg lettuce wraps to make up the fajitas.

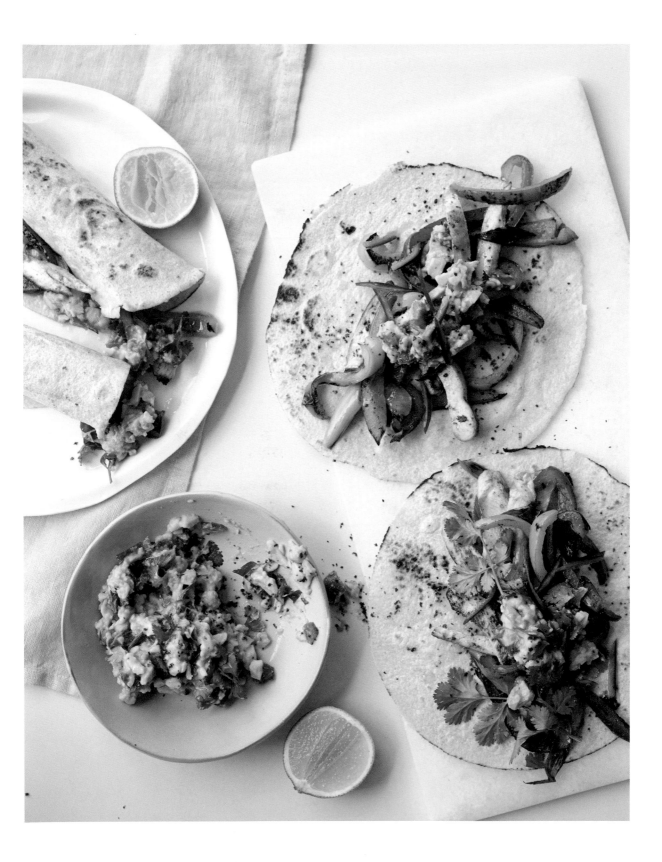

oh my cod

345 CALORIES / 31G CARBS / 13G FAT / 30G PROTEIN

Three words you want to hear when you cook this delicious fish and chips takeaway alternative. Oh My Cod!

serves 2

1½ large sweet potatoes, cut into chips (I like chunky wedges)
1 tablespoon melted coconut oil, plus a little extra
¼ teaspoon black pepper
1 teaspoon Italian seasoning
a pinch of salt
300–400g cod loin, or your favourite white fish
80g frozen peas
a pinch of chilli powder
1 teaspoon finely chopped flat-leaf parsley
1 teaspoon finely chopped mint

Preheat the oven to 180°C/gas mark 4 and pop in a baking tray lined with baking parchment to heat.

Tip the sweet potato wedges into a large bowl and add the coconut oil and seasoning, then mix to coat the wedges well. Spread the wedges out on the heated baking tray and roast for 25–30 minutes until soft.

Put the fish on a baking tray or in a baking dish, cover with foil and cook for 15–20 minutes.

Cook the peas in a pan of boiling water for 4–5 minutes, or according to the packet instructions. Transfer one-third of the peas into a bowl and mash them with a fork.

Heat a frying pan with a little coconut oil and add the chilli, then the parsley and mint.

Add the mashed peas and cooked whole peas and stir well. Heat through and serve alongside the fish and sweet potato wedges.

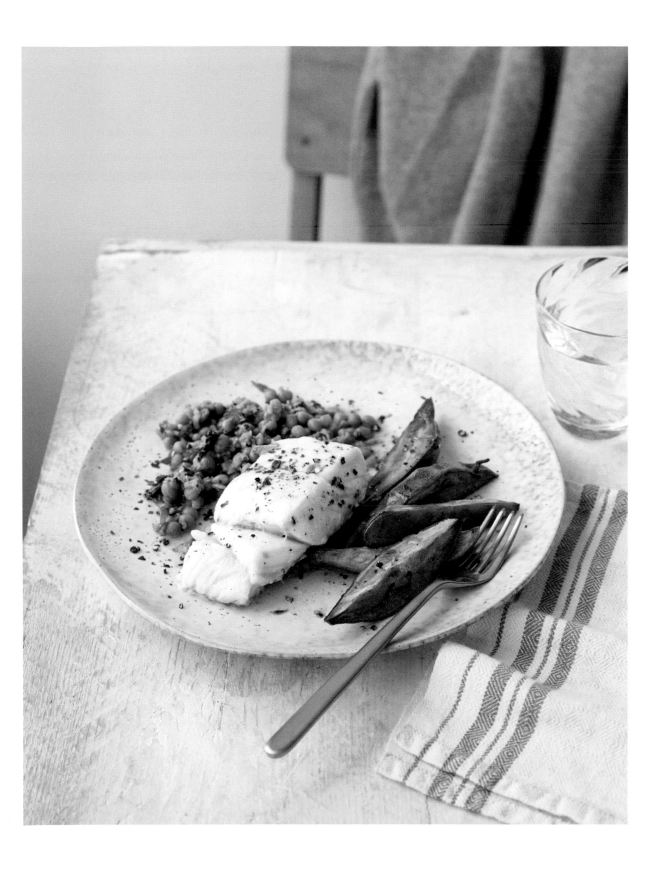

chicken on a stick

173 CALORIES / 0.3G CARBS / 7G FAT / 29G PROTEIN

If it comes on a stick, you know it's good! Candy floss, Magnums, cocktail sausages... and this healthy chicken option doesn't let the team down! Full of lean protein and great flavour.

serves 4

1 tablespoon lemon juice
2 teaspoons dried oregano
1 tablespoon olive oil
1 garlic clove, crushed
4 skinless chicken breast fillets
   (about 550g), cut into cubes
salt and freshly ground black
   pepper
mixed leaves, to serve

Combine the lemon juice with the oregano, oil, garlic and salt and pepper in a small jar and shake. Pour this over the chicken, massaging it into the chunks with your hands. Cover and chill in the fridge for 2 hours to marinate.

Thread the chicken cubes onto eight metal or wooden skewers and cook under a hot grill for 20 minutes, turning them after 10 minutes, until cooked all the way through and the flesh has turned from pink to white.

Serve with some mixed leaves on the side.

this chick's shredded

387 CALORIES / 32G CARBS / 14G FAT / 34G PROTEIN

When you have that 'I just crushed my workout' kinda vibe going, shred that chicken, because we know that true healthcare starts in the kitchen.

Preheat the oven to 180°C/gas mark 4.

Put the chicken breast on a baking tray and roast in the oven for 30 minutes. Shred the chicken into tiny pieces and leave to cool.

Cook the quinoa according to packet instructions, then leave to cool.

To make the dressing, whisk all the ingredients together in a small bowl. Refrigerate until ready to serve.

Combine the spinach, mixed leaves and cabbage together in a large salad bowl. Add the almonds to the bowl with the cranberries.

Add the cooled chicken and quinoa to the salad bowl. Toss to combine, then pour over the dressing, toss again and serve.

serves 1

1 skinless chicken breast fillet
50g quinoa
20g baby spinach
30g mixed leaves
75g red cabbage, finely sliced
6 almonds, finely chopped
15g dried cranberries

FOR THE DRESSING
1 tablespoon finely chopped
   flat-leaf parsley
1 teaspoon extra virgin olive
   oil
1 teaspoon water
1 teaspoon honey
1 teaspoon lemon juice
salt, to taste

Protein is the most weight-loss friendly macronutrient and can drastically reduce appetite and cravings

——

daddy's dinner

527 CALS / 56G CARBS / 13G FAT / 45G PROTEIN

A girl's first love is her daddy, and how could you not love the man who makes you this classic on a cold winter evening? It's like a huge hug on a plate.

serves 2–3

550g sweet potatoes, peeled and
    diced
1 tablespoon coconut oil
2 carrots, peeled and cut into
    batons
1 large onion or spring onion
    (green parts only), chopped
2 garlic cloves, chopped
550g lean 5% fat Irish beef mince
1 tablespoon tomato purée
5 tablespoons red wine
2 tablespoons Worcestershire
    sauce
300ml hot beef stock
1 tablespoon plain flour
a few sprigs of thyme
    teaspoon grated nutmeg
salt and freshly ground black
    pepper, to taste

Preheat the oven to 200°C/gas mark 6.

Add the sweet potatoes to a pan of boiling water and cook for about 20 minutes until soft.

Meanwhile, heat a large frying pan over a medium heat and melt the coconut oil. Add the carrots to the frying pan and stir to make sure they are all coated in oil.

Add the onion and garlic to the carrots, stir to mix, then increase the heat slightly and cook all the vegetables until they are a nice golden brown colour.

Add the mince to the pan, season with salt and black pepper and cook until completely browned. Stir in the tomato purée and cook for 1 minute. Pour in the red wine, increase the heat and bring to the boil for about 30 seconds–1 minute to allow the liquid to reduce. Add the Worcestershire sauce, boil and allow to reduce for another minute. Pour in the beef stock and add the flour, stirring until it is completely mixed in, then add the thyme. There should be a decent bit of liquid in the pan, so let the juice reduce to your desired thickness.

By this stage the sweet potatoes should be ready, so drain and mash them in a bowl. Season with salt, black pepper and the nutmeg.

Pour the beef mix into a large ovenproof dish and shake the dish from side to side to get a nice even layer. Top with the mashed sweet potatoes and style to your desire – I like to make small mountains on mine. Transfer to the oven and cook for 15 minutes.

After the 15 minutes, remove the dish from the oven and leave it to sit for 5–10 minutes. Once the dish has cooled, it's time to serve and enjoy.

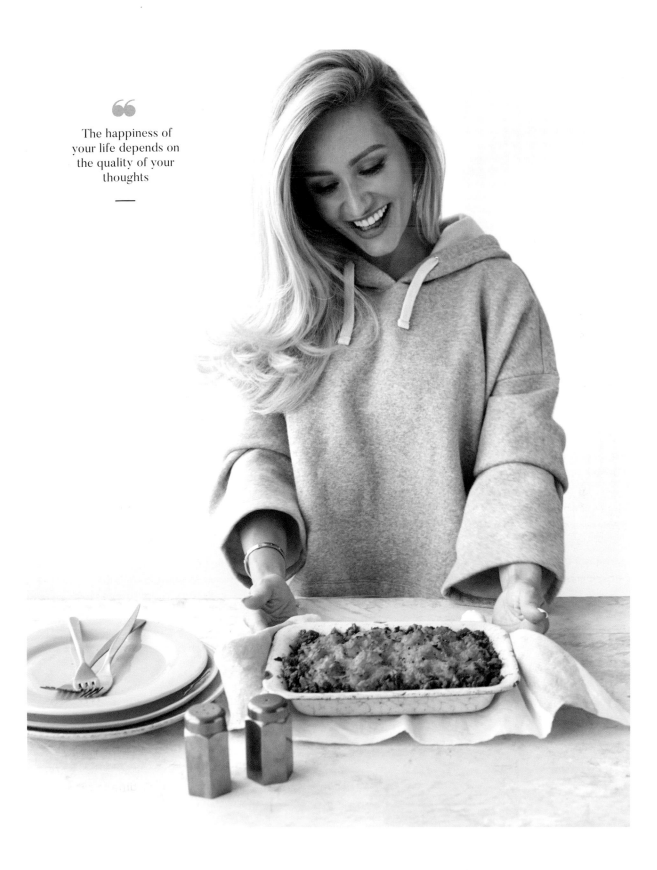

slaw monster burger & fries

501 CALORIES / 22G CARBS / 23G FAT / 53G PROTEIN (BURGER, FRIES AND SLAW)

This is my version of the ultimate comfort food – chicken burger and coleslaw. Try to cut all your fries the same size and not too large, so that they cook at the same rate, and be wary of adding salt or seasonings with added salt as these draw moisture from the fries and create steam which equals soggy fries!

serves 4

800g lean turkey mince
1 egg, beaten
1 tablespoon extra virgin olive oil
1 small shallot, chopped
1 garlic clove, minced
1 teaspoon dried oregano
80g lettuce, shredded
2 tomatoes, sliced

FOR THE SWEET POTATO FRIES

2 large sweet potatoes, cut into
   5mm thick slices
1–2 tablespoons coconut oil, melted
seasoning of choice

FOR THE SLAW

½ red cabbage, shredded
2 medium carrots, grated
15g flat-leaf parsley, chopped
120g vegan mayonnaise
1 tablespoon apple cider vinegar
1 tablespoon Dijon mustard
½ teaspoon celery seeds
squeeze of lemon (optional)
salt and freshly ground black
   pepper, to taste

Preheat the oven to 180°C/gas mark 4. Line a baking tray with greaseproof paper and pop it in the oven to heat.

In a large bowl, mix the sweet potato fries with the coconut oil. Add a little seasoning as the oil will help the spices stick to the sweet potatoes. Evenly arrange the fries on the preheated baking tray and bake for 40 minutes. You will need to turn them halfway through to ensure that all sides are cooked.

Combine the turkey, egg, oil, shallot and garlic in a bowl. Mix well and shape into four patties. Season the patties with the oregano and some black pepper. Place under the grill and cook for 10 minutes, turning them over after 5 minutes.

Meanwhile, make the slaw. Combine the cabbage, carrots and parsley into a big bowl.

In a separate bowl, stir together the mayo, vinegar, mustard and celery seeds and season with salt and black pepper – sometimes I add a squeeze of lemon. Pour the dressing over the shredded slaw veggies and mix well.

When the patties are cooked through, serve topped with lettuce and tomatoes and the fries and slaw alongside.

tip I just top my burgers with lettuce and tomato as I find red onion can cause bloating. Another alternative is to add 60ml vegan mayonnaise and 60ml dairy-free yogurt to the slaw instead of vegan mayo.

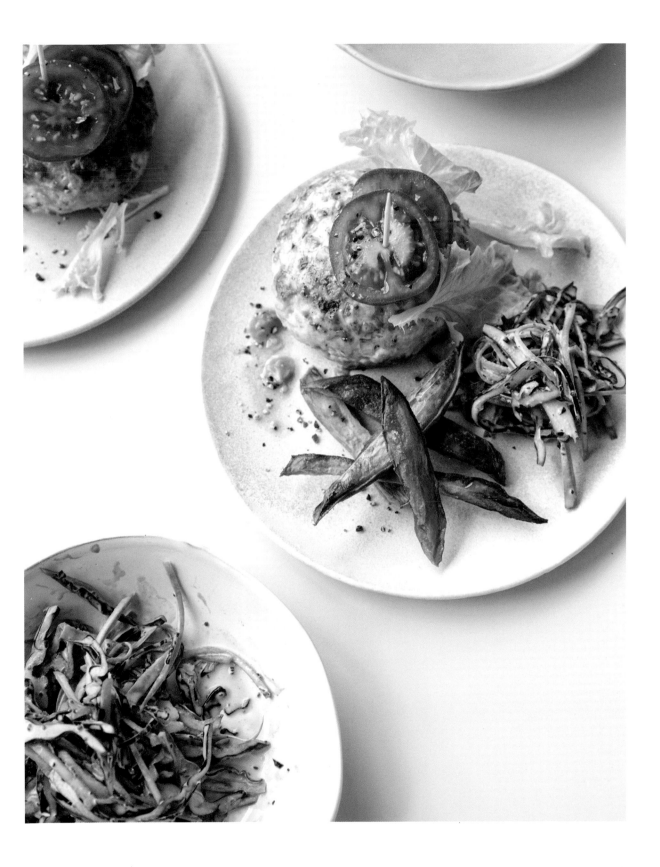

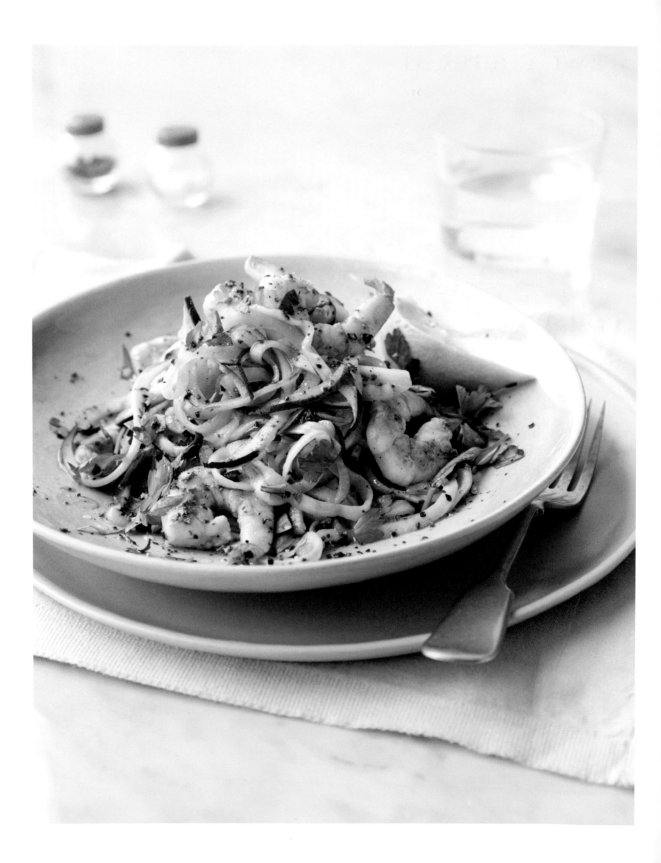

prawn courgetti

213 CALS / 4G CARBS / 10G FAT / 21G PROTEIN

What the health? Spaghetti that won't make you bloat, yes, it's true, and this recipe is also super filling and delicious.

Place a large frying pan over a medium heat. Add the oil and heat it for 1 minute, then add the chilli flakes and cook for 1 minute, stirring constantly. Add the prawns and cook for about 3 minutes, stirring as needed, until they are cooked through and have turned pink. Season the prawns with salt and black pepper and then, using a slotted spoon, transfer them to a bowl, leaving any liquid in the pan.

Add the wine and lemon juice to the pan. Using a wooden spoon, scrape any brown bits from the bottom of the pan and cook the liquid for 2 minutes.

Add the courgettes and cook, stirring occasionally, for 2 minutes.

Return the prawns to the pan and toss to combine. Season with salt and black pepper, garnish with the parsley and serve immediately.

serves 2

1½ tablespoons olive oil
¼ teaspoon chilli flakes
200g raw king prawns, peeled
70ml white wine
2 tablespoons lemon juice
2 courgettes (about 350g), spiralised
salt and freshly ground black pepper, to taste
20g flat-leaf parsley, chopped, to serve

tropical tuna

418 CALORIES / 14G CARBS / 22G FAT / 43G PROTEIN

Aloha! Is summer coming, have you been beachwear shopping, are you feeling in a tropical state of mind? So clean, so lean, so fresh, this tuna dish is a taste of paradise.

serves 1

150–200g tuna steak
1 teaspoon sesame seeds
1 teaspoon olive oil
juice of 1 lime
30g spinach
salt and freshly ground black
   pepper, to taste

FOR THE SALSA
1 tomato
½ avocado
100g papaya
1 jalapeño chilli
15g coriander, roughly chopped
squeeze of lime juice

To make the salsa, dice the tomato, avocado, papaya and chilli, mix well in a small bowl and stir in the coriander. Season with salt and a squeeze of fresh lime.

Place the tuna on a plate and season with salt and black pepper. Sprinkle half the sesame seeds on one side of the tuna, patting them onto the tuna steak, then repeat on the other side.

Heat the oil in a griddle pan over a high heat until smoking. Add the tuna and cook for 2 minutes on each side, or until cooked to your liking.

Place a frying pan over a medium heat, then add the spinach. It's OK to pile it up a bit, as it will wilt quickly, but even so, it may not all fit in at first. Using tongs, gently toss and turn the spinach so that all the unwilted leaves make contact with the bottom of the pan.

To serve, put the spinach onto a serving plate and place the tuna on top. Spoon the salsa on the side.

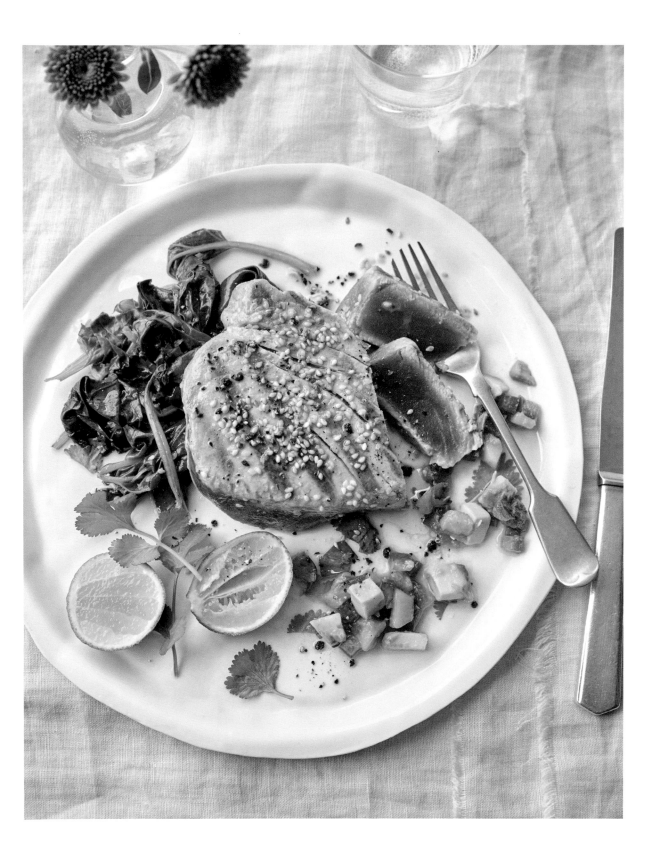

talking tacos

270 CALORIES / 9.5G CARBS / 4.6G FAT / 25.5G PROTEIN (EXCLUDING TACOS)

Make your way up the beach to the promenade and order some of these Californian-inspired fish tacos. Me and my brothers love surfer food and we live on it when we're hitting up the waves (well, they do, you'll find me on a beach bed working on my tan). This recipe is vibrant, fresh and super light, which means you can eat it over and over again and still get back in the water.

serves 4

2 garlic cloves, crushed

juice of 1 lime

⅔ teaspoon ground cumin

¼ teaspoon chilli flakes

500g skinless white fish fillets, such as cod

fresh lettuce leaves or corn tortillas (optional), to serve

FOR THE SALSA

20g coriander sprigs

3 garlic cloves

2 tablespoons lime juice

2 jalapeño chillies, roughly chopped

½ onion, roughly chopped

5 tomatoes, roughly chopped

1½ teaspoons ground cumin

a pinch of salt

FOR THE GUACAMOLE

2 avocados, halved and stoned

1 tomato, diced and seeds removed

juice of 3 limes

a large handful of finely chopped coriander

1 tablespoon Frank's hot sauce (optional)

salt and freshly ground black pepper, to taste

Combine the garlic, lime juice, cumin and chilli flakes in a dish, then add the fish and leave to marinate for 15 minutes.

Preheat the oven to 180°C/gas mark 4.

Transfer the fish and marinade to a baking tray and bake for 20 minutes, or until the fish is cooked through. Once cooked, flake into a serving dish.

To make the salsa, add all the ingredients to a food processor or NutriBullet. Blitz until the ingredients are diced – careful not to overdo it – you want a chunky salsa, not a soupy salsa. Scoop into a bowl and season to taste.

To make the guacamole, scoop the avocado flesh into a bowl and mash it up with a fork. Add the remaining ingredients and mix well. Taste for seasoning.

Serve the fish on fresh lettuce leaves or lightly baked tortillas and top with a little salsa and/or guacamole.

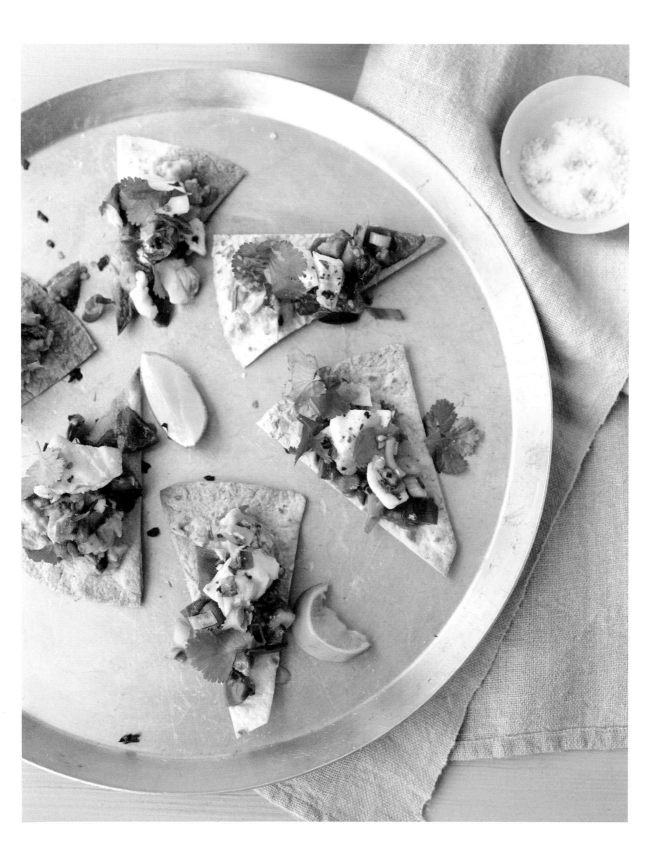

señorita salmon

473 CALORIES / 29.4G CARBS / 26G FAT / 31.9G PROTEIN

Don't you just love being on vacation and not knowing what day it is?! Take Señorita salmon on your vacation for a fresh, light evening delight.

serves 2

1 tablespoon lime juice, plus
　zest of 1 lime
1 garlic clove, crushed
2 skinless salmon fillets
salt and freshly ground black
　pepper

FOR THE MANGO SALSA

½ mango, peeled, stoned and
　chopped into small pieces
½ red pepper, chopped into small
　pieces
1 tablespoon chopped coriander
¼ avocado, halved, stoned, peeled
　and chopped into small pieces
1 teaspoon lime juice
½ teaspoon olive oil

FOR THE COCONUT RICE

100g brown rice, cooked
200ml light coconut milk
1 teaspoon coconut flakes

In a deep baking dish, mix together the lime juice, zest, garlic and a little salt and black pepper to make the salmon marinade. Place salmon in the dish and spoon the marinade over the top, Cover and chill for 15–20 minutes, turning halfway through.

While the salmon is marinating, prepare the coconut rice. Put the rice, coconut milk and coconut flakes in a medium saucepan and bring to the boil. Cover and simmer for about 15 minutes until all the liquid has been absorbed. Drain off the excess liquid if necessary, fluff up the rice with a fork and leave it to rest for 5 minutes.

Preheat the grill to medium. In a medium bowl, mix together all the mango salsa ingredients.

Grill the salmon for 3 minutes on each side, or until cooked through. Serve topped with the mango salsa and the coconut rice on the side.

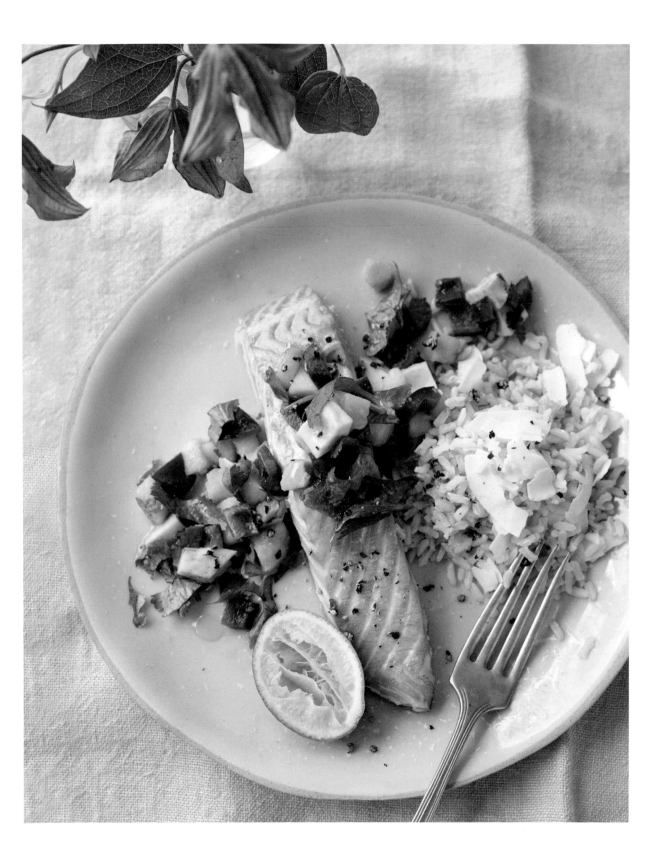

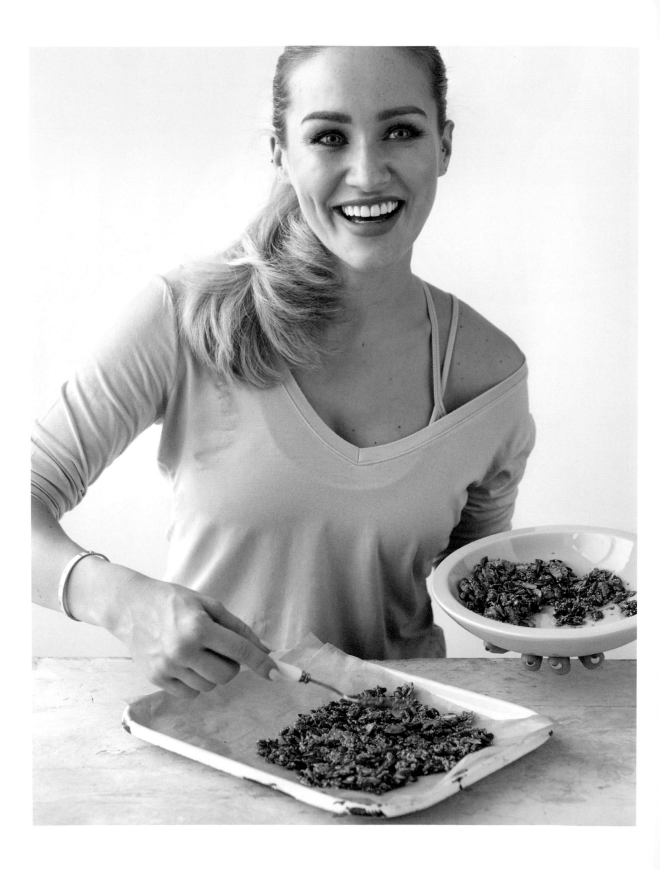

snacks

guac & sticks

144 CALORIES / 2G CARBS / 14G FAT / 2G PROTEIN (GUACAMOLE)

You can buy so many pre-cut veggie crudités in your local supermarket, but I find it's cheaper to buy the whole veg and make your own. I peel my cucumber when cutting it up, because the skin makes me a little bloated, but that's up to you.

V

serves 4

2 avocados, halved and stoned

1 tomato, finely diced

3 tablespoons finely chopped coriander

2 tablespoons lime juice

a pinch of salt

a pinch of cayenne pepper

1 teaspoon Frank's hot sauce (optional)

200g carrot batons

½ cucumber, peeled and cut into batons

1 red pepper, deseeded and cut into strips

Scoop the avocado flesh into a mixing bowl, then mash it up until smooth or all the big chunks are broken up. Add the tomato, coriander, lime juice and salt. Taste and adjust the seasoning accordingly – sometimes I add a little more lime juice. Mix to your preferred guacamole consistency.

Transfer to a serving bowl and dust with the cayenne pepper. If you want some extra spice, add a little splash of Frank's hot sauce.

Serve the guac in a bowl in the centre of a serving platter with the chopped vegetables all around it.

 tip How do you know when an avocado is ripe and ready? Pop off the stem at the top of the avocado: if what's revealed is bright green, the avocado is ripe and ready to be eaten; if it's brown, you're likely to find brown spots on the flesh.

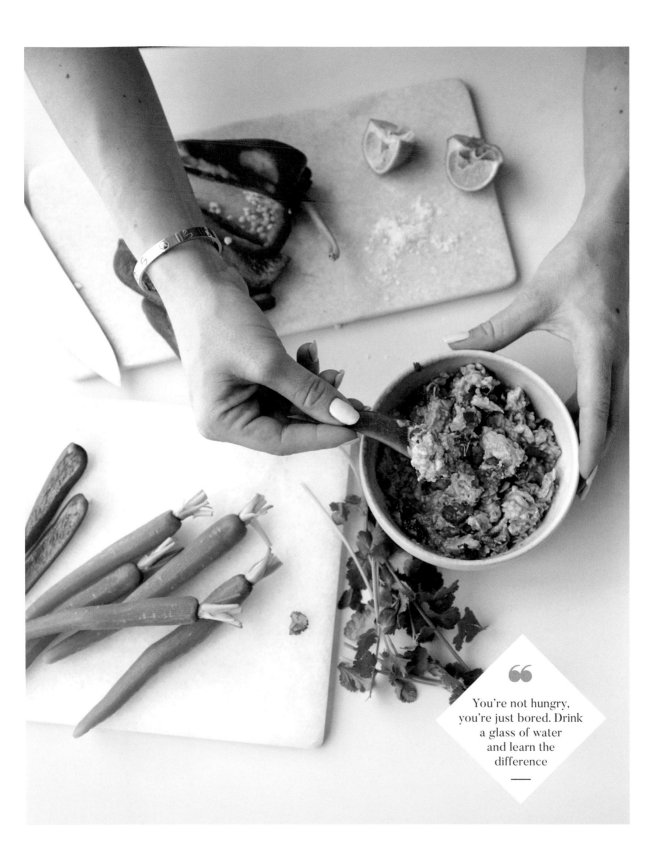

> **"**
> You're not hungry,
> you're just bored. Drink
> a glass of water
> and learn the
> difference
> —

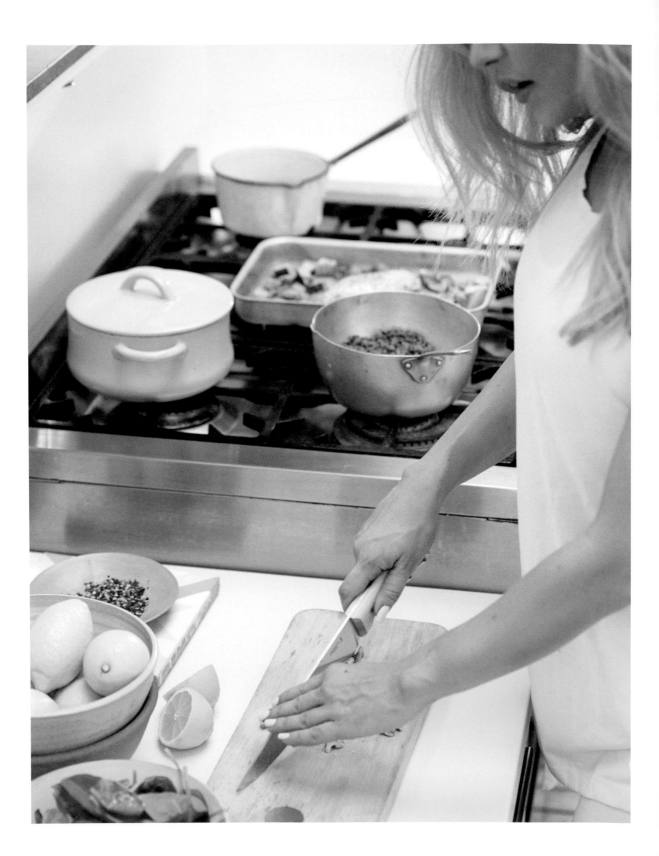

hunky chunky hummus

230 CALORIES / 16G CARBS / 14G FAT / 10.5G PROTEIN

The secret to perfectly smooth, creamy hummus is removing the chickpea skins before blitzing. Chickpeas are high in iron folate and vitamin B, which are essential nutrients for those following a vegan or vegetarian lifestyle. Enjoy with some delicious chunky veg as a delicious appetiser or afternoon snack. Choose coconut yogurt for a vegan option.

serves 4

Soak the chickpeas in at least double the volume of water. When you are ready to make the hummus, drain the chickpeas in a sieve and rinse under cold running water. Rub the chickpeas to remove the skins (see Tip).

Put the lemon juice and seasoning in a food processor and blitz together with the tahini and garlic. Add the chickpeas, olive oil and yogurt, and blend until smooth and creamy. Serve at room temperature with a drizzle of oil and sprinkle over the paprika.

Slice the celery sticks lengthways into three pieces. Then cut them down the centre so you have six pieces. I eat my green beans crunchy, so grab a handful and add them to the serving platter along with the carrots, cucumber and radishes.

Serve the hummus in the centre of a serving platter and enjoy this crunchy dipping snack with the crudités.

400g can chickpeas, drained
    and rinsed
juice of 1 lemon
½ teaspoon salt
½ teaspoon freshly ground
    black pepper
4 tablespoons tahini
2 garlic cloves, peeled
2 teaspoons olive oil, plus
    extra for drizzling
2 tablespoons plain yogurt of your
    choice
1 teaspoon paprika

FOR THE CRUDITÉS
2 celery sticks
75g green beans
200g carrots, scrubbed and cut
    into batons
½ cucumber, peeled and cut into
    batons
8 radishes, scrubbed

tip   You don't have to remove the skins of the chickpeas, but it will make your hummus silky smooth.

oh she glows
papaya & turmeric chia pots

228 CALORIES / 14G CARBS / 14G FAT / 7G PROTEIN

Mixed with a blend of beauty-boosting ingredients, Oh she Glows is a tropical treat, which is just as beautiful as it is delicious. Stay golden all day long.

V

serves 4

350ml unsweetened almond or coconut milk, plus extra (optional)
1 teaspoon honey or stevia
1 teaspoon vanilla extract
½ teaspoon ground cinnamon
½ mango, peeled, stoned and roughly chopped
1 teaspoon ground turmeric
6 tablespoons chia seeds
1 papaya, cut into small chunks
80g raspberries
25g pistachios, chopped

Blend the milk, honey or stevia, vanilla, cinnamon, mango and turmeric in a blender until smooth.

Put the chia seeds in a bowl and pour over the smoothie mixture. Stir and set aside. Stir again 5 minutes later to prevent the seeds sticking together. Transfer to an airtight container, mix in the small chunks of papaya and refrigerate. Leave to thicken for 2 hours or overnight if possible.

When you are ready to serve, add extra milk if the texture looks too thick. Spoon into glasses and top with the raspberries and pistachios.

tip The chia seed mix will keep for 3–4 days in the fridge in an airtight container.

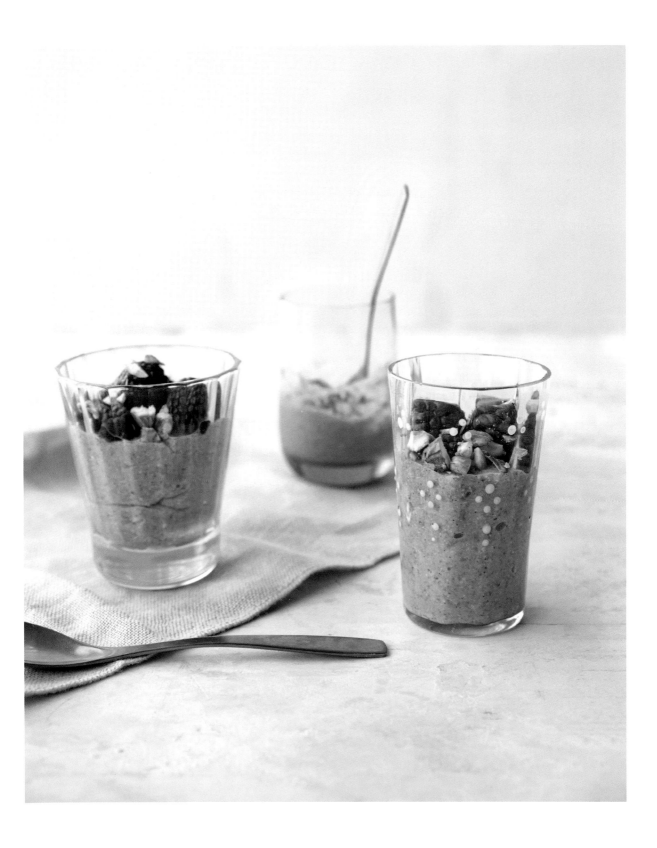

crusher cookies

59 CALORIES / 2G CARBS / 14G FAT / 7G PROTEIN (PER COOKIE)

Crush those cravings with Crusher cookies. This crunchy recipe is the perfect combo of sweet and salty, which will give you a proper boost of vitamins, minerals and omega oils to power you through the day. Perfect for vegans and vegetarians, too.

V

makes 12

20g coconut oil
1 tablespoon maple syrup
1 teaspoon maca powder
35g ground flaxseed
25g sunflower seeds
30g pumpkin seeds
10g flaked almonds
20g chia seeds

Preheat the oven to 110°C/gas mark ¼. Line a medium-sized ovenproof dish with parchment paper.

Melt the coconut oil in a pan over a low heat. Add the maple syrup and maca powder and whisk well. Add the remaining ingredients and mix together. Tip the mixture onto the prepared dish and spread it out evenly.

Now for the long part, but it's oh so worth it for the sweet crunchiness. Pop the mixture in the oven to slow-toast for 6 hours. After 3 hours, remove from the oven, place on a chopping board and cut into cookie rounds using cutters about 2.5cm in diameter. Turn the cookies over and pop them back into the oven for the remaining 3 hours.

Leave in the dish until cool enough to handle, then transfer to a wire rack to cool completely. You can keep the cookies in an airtight container for up to a week.

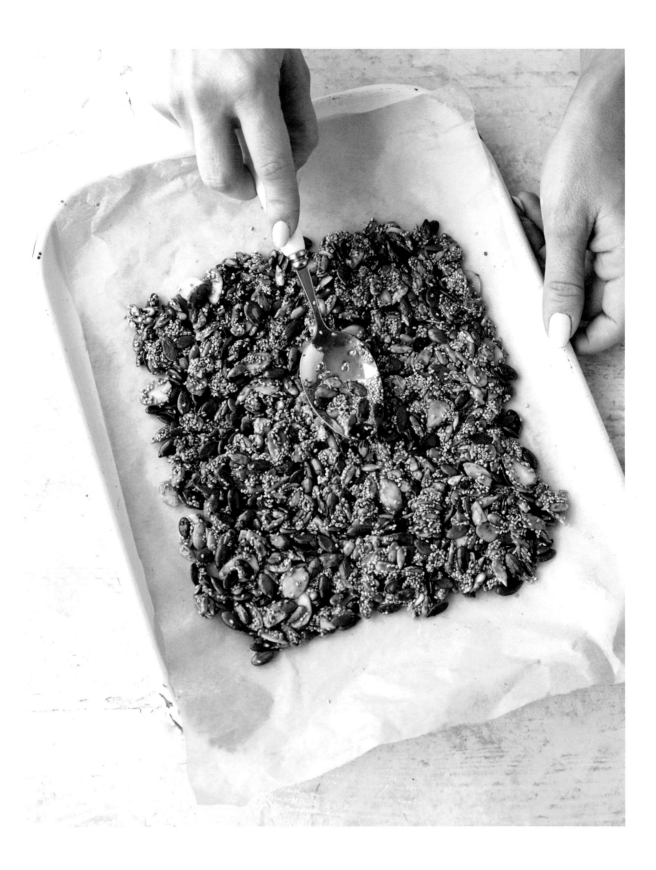

loco coco

318 CALORIES / 12G CARBS / 28G FAT / 8G PROTEIN

This is one of my favourite go-to puddings, especially in the evening. Cinnamon naturally helps balance sugar cravings by controlling blood glucose levels.

serves 1

75g mixed berries, such as
blueberries, strawberries and
raspberries
100g coconut yogurt
1 tablespoon almond butter
½ peach, sliced
1 teaspoon ground cinnamon

Pop the berries in a bowl and microwave on high for 30 seconds.

Add the yogurt to a bowl and swirl in the almond butter. Top with the hot berries, add the peach slices and dust with the cinnamon.

berry bountiful

228 CALORIES / 16G CARBS / 17G FAT / 3G PROTEIN

If you want a quick spring-summer dessert that doesn't require cooking, then look no further – the only planning you need is putting the coconut cream/milk in the fridge overnight.

serves 4

400ml can coconut cream or milk
½ teaspoon vanilla extract
(optional)
1 tablespoon coconut sugar or
maple syrup
600g mixed berries, such as
blueberries, strawberries and
raspberries

Chill the coconut cream or milk in the fridge overnight – be sure not to shake or let anyone move the can while it's cooling.

The next day, chill a large mixing bowl in the fridge for 10 minutes. Remove the coconut cream or milk from the fridge and remove the lid. Scrape out the thickened cream on top, leaving the liquid behind. Spoon the hardened cream into your chilled mixing bowl. Beat for 30 seconds with a mixer, then add the vanilla and sweetener and mix until for about a minute until creamy and smooth.

Use immediately or refrigerate – it will harden and set in the fridge the longer it's chilled. Spoon into bowls and top with mixed berries.

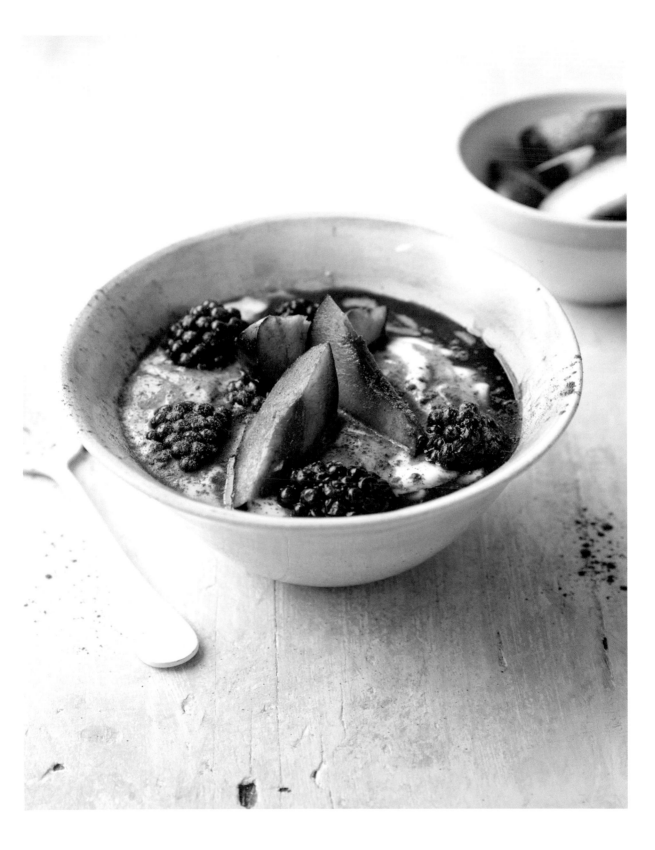

no pudge fudge

96 CALORIES / 1G CARBS / 9G FAT / 2.5G PROTEIN (PER 15G PIECE)

Sweet, gooey deliciousness. Fudge has always been a Madden family favourite. We are all a little coconut crazy these days, and my nutty treat will satisfy any sweet craving.

serves 6

120g almond butter
2½ tablespoons virgin coconut oil
 or 30g coconut butter
2½ tablespoons liquid sweetener
 of choice (optional)
a few drops maple extract
 (optional)
sprinkle of pink salt

Heat a saucepan over a medium heat and add the almond butter and coconut oil or butter. Gently warm until they have both melted, then add your choice of sweetener, if using, and mix well.

Spoon the liquid fudge into an ice-cube tray or freezable sweets mould (I use ice-cube trays). Sprinkle a little salt on top and transfer to the freezer for a few hours until solid. Surprisingly, these don't take as long to freeze as you may think.

Pop them out of the moulds and eat immediately.

awesome almonds

195 CALORIES / 2G CARBS / 18G FAT / 6G PROTEIN

Of all tree nuts, almonds rank the highest in protein, vitamin E, fibre and calcium, so I always have a pot in my bag to snack on when I'm on the go. The sweetness of the maple and spice of the cinnamon makes this version a great mid-afternoon snack.

serves 10

300g whole almonds
1 tablespoon coconut oil
1 teaspoon ground cinnamon
1 teaspoon sea salt
1 teaspoon maple syrup

Preheat the oven to 180°C/gas mark 4 and line a large baking tray with baking paper.

Spread the nuts in a single layer over a baking tray and toast in the oven for 10 minutes.

Heat the coconut oil, cinnamon, salt and maple syrup in a saucepan over a low heat until melted. Remove from the heat and pour over the nuts, mixing until they are all covered. Leave to cool and enjoy.

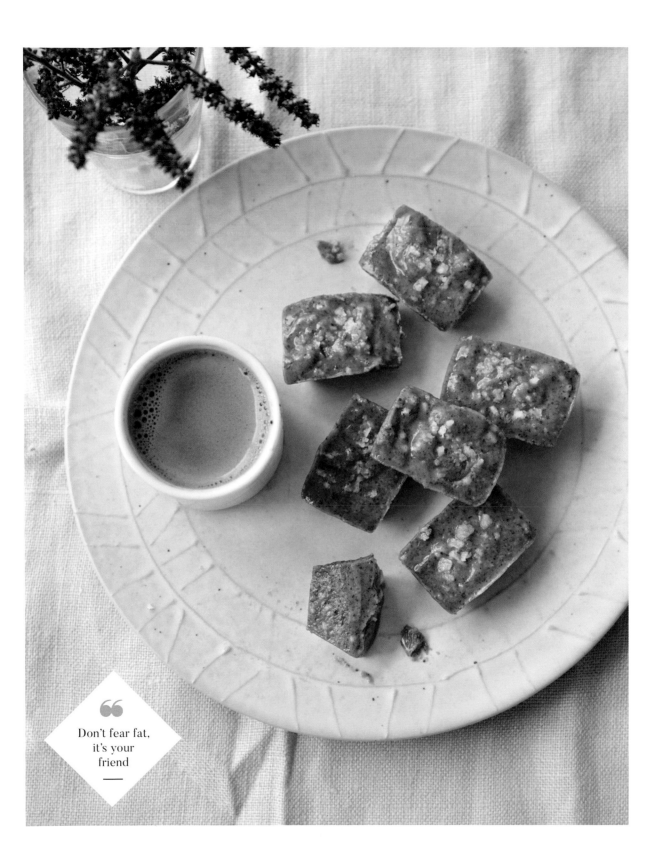

66

Don't fear fat,
it's your
friend

—

mint mountain milkshake

305 CALORIES / 17G CARBS / 22G FAT / 9G PROTEIN

Did someone say MILKSHAKE?? YAAAAS... Who knew plants could go into milkshakes and still taste delicious? My dreamy dark-chocolate-chip Mint Mountain is the perfect sweet, innocent indulgence when craving a treat. With fresh mint leaves it really is a cool breeze. When your milkshake is bloat free, damn right it's better than yours.

serves 2

180g coconut yogurt
1 tablespoon maple syrup
250ml almond milk
a handful of ice
3-4 mint leaves
40g dark chocolate chips
30g baby spinach

Put all the ingredients into a blender, starting with the wet ingredients first so that the dry ingredients don't stick to the sides. Blitz until smooth. Pour and serve.

shlomocha

150 CALORIES / 5G CARBS / 5G FAT / 18G PROTEIN

Like many people, my coffee habit started with the sweet and sugary frappuccino. Bad news: they are full of sugar and dairy – bloatastic. Good news: I came up with my own version. This is a quick and easy way to bring your favourite ice-cold frappuccino drinks home. No need for that over-priced coffee run now. Winning.

V

serves 1

120ml almond milk
120ml cold brew coffee
1 shot of espresso
a handful of ice
1 teaspoon cocoa powder
20g scoop of vegan vanilla protein powder

Put all the ingredients into a blender, starting with the wet ingredients first so that the dry ingredients don't stick to the sides. Blitz until smooth. Pour and serve.

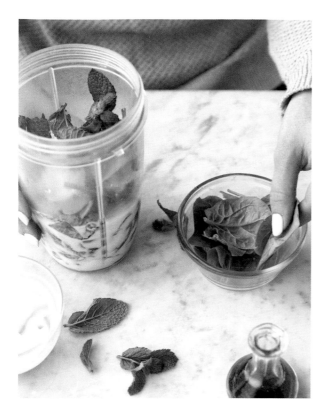

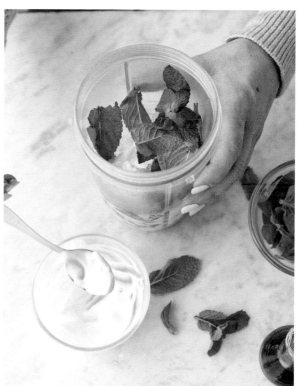

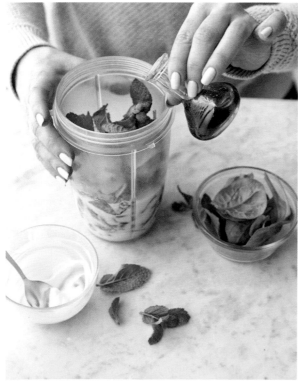

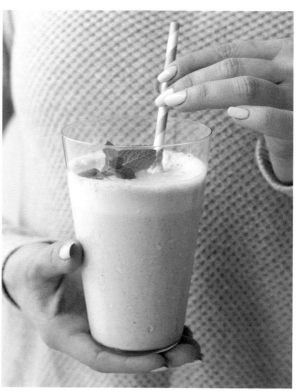

crunchy monkey ice cream

394 CALORIES / 55G CARBS / 16G FAT / 9G PROTEIN

Deliciously chunky, banana-chocolatey-chip ice cream without the cream. How? This is made with sweet, ripe bananas, almond milk and chocolatey goodness so you will have to keep reminding yourself it's dairy and sugar free.

serves 2

5 overripe bananas, sliced and
   frozen
100ml almond milk
1 teaspoon vanilla bean paste
30g cocoa nibs
25g mixed nuts, such as pistachios,
   almonds or Brazil nuts, crushed

In two separate mixers, blend half the frozen banana, half the milk and half the vanilla bean paste until smooth. Transfer to a bowl and stir in cocoa nibs.

Top with mixed nuts and serve immediately.

angel delight

219 CALORIES / 20G CARBS / 15G FAT / 3G PROTEIN

Papaya is packed with numerous health benefits including aiding digestion. With its sweet, soft, butter-like taste, this exotic fruit is wonderful for curbing those sweet cravings.

serves 2

1 papaya
2 tablespoons coconut yogurt
1 teaspoon bee pollen
2 lime wedges

Cut the papaya in half and scoop out the weird black ball seeds. Divide the yogurt among the holes in each papaya half. Top with the bee pollen and squeeze the lime wedges over the top.

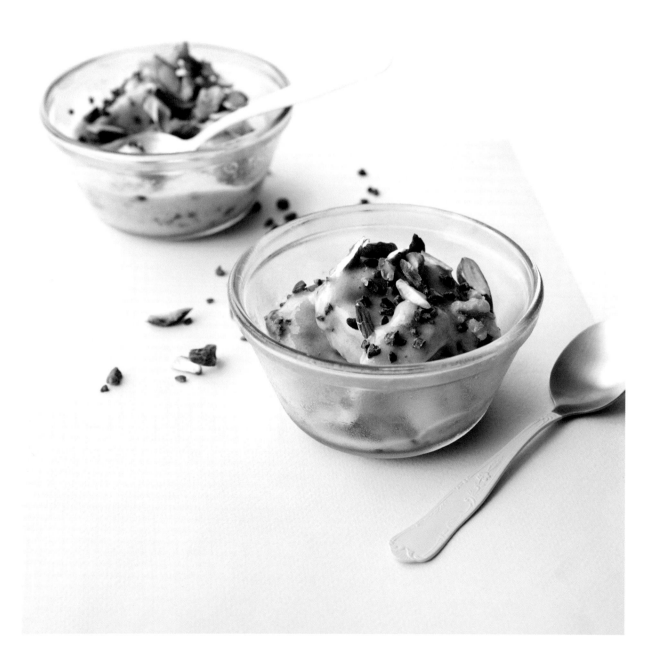

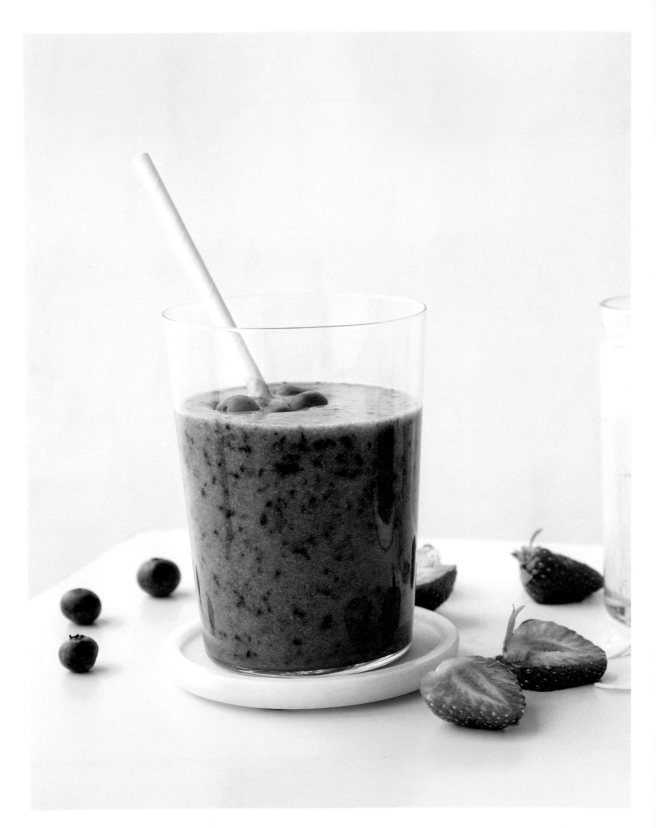

drinks

200g pineapple, roughly
  chopped
200g blueberries
75g strawberries, hulled
½ medium banana, roughly
  chopped
250ml nut milk, such as almond
  milk

berrly legal

This combo of ingredients makes a perfectly smooth-tasting smoothie. I sometimes replace the strawberries with raspberries to give it a bit more zing. Pineapple creates a tropical, smooth and creamy base.

Add all the ingredients to a blender and blitz until smooth. Pour into two glasses and enjoy.

serves 2

250ml strong coffee
½ banana, chopped
30g gluten-free rolled oats
1 teaspoon raw organic cacao
  powder
1 tablespoon flaxseed
⅛ teaspoon ground cinnamon
250ml nut milk, such as almond
1 teaspoon maca powder
¼ teaspoon stevia or raw organic
  vanilla

dan-delion

Getting to the gym can sometimes be the hardest part of the workout. Need a pre-workout smoothie to pep you up? Then it's time to Dan-delion. Not only is this sweet and flavoursome, the added coffee gives you that caffeine kick, too. Drink it, then crush it.

Add all the ingredients to a blender and blitz until smooth. Pour into two glasses and enjoy.

serves 2

250ml coconut water
75g pineapple chunks
100g spinach
1 banana, roughly chopped
1 teaspoon maca powder
½ teaspoon camu camu powder

the cure

Popping bottles or you've had one gin and slimline tonic too many? Don't worry, I come bearing good news. This is one nutritious, smooth formula to help boost your body and mind. So refresh and restore with this green and citrus combo.

Add all the ingredients to a blender and blitz until smooth. Pour into two glasses and enjoy.

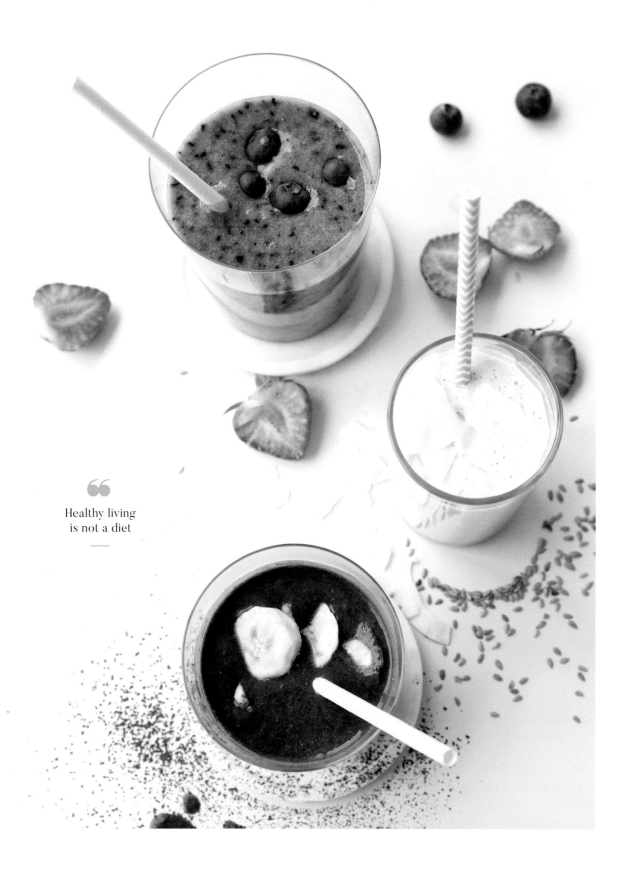

> Healthy living
> is not a diet

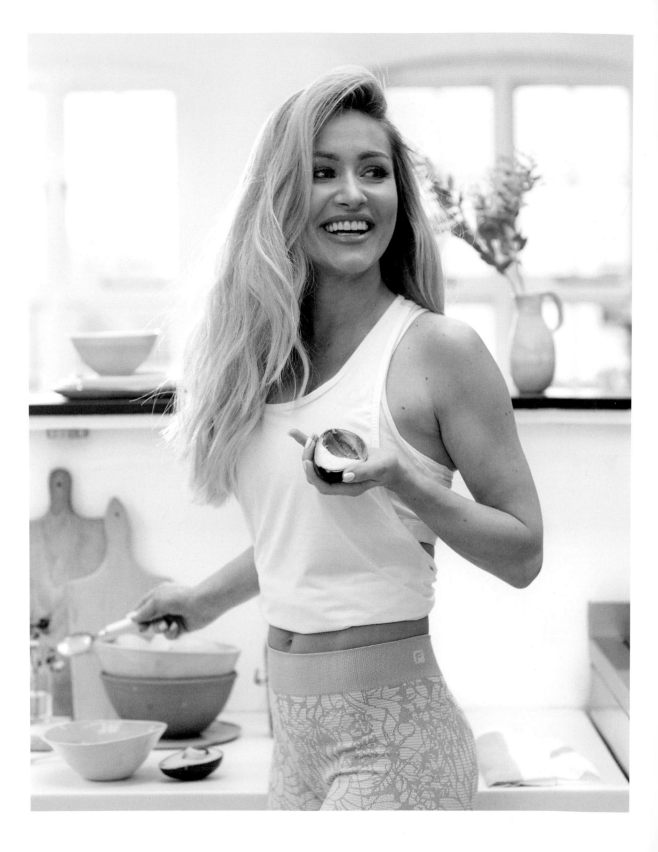

wired

The perfect formula to support peak performance, stamina and longevity, while aiding in healthy recovery. Avocado makes this smoothie not only creamier, it also adds healthy fats for a balanced diet.

Add all the ingredients to a blender and blitz until smooth. Pour into two glasses and enjoy.

serves 2

250ml chilled green tea
60g spinach
½ cucumber, peeled and roughly chopped
200g pineapple, roughly chopped
juice of 1 lemon
½ avocado, roughly chopped
1 tablespoon freshly grated ginger
a handful of coriander

into the wild

All the ingredients taste as if you've picked them fresh from your garden, and they blend perfectly together. The combination of spinach and flaxseeds supplies any healthy diet with additional and beneficial fibre, which is important to keep the digestive system in shape.

Add all the ingredients to a blender and blitz until smooth. Pour into a glass and enjoy.

serves 1

a handful of spinach leaves
1.5cm piece of fresh ginger, peeled and grated
1 teaspoon flaxseeds
a handful of kale
2 teaspoons chia seeds
¼ cucumber, peeled and roughly chopped
½ teaspoon chlorella
¼ avocado, halved, stoned and roughly chopped
70ml water

morning glory

Another glorious morning smoothie packed with hormone-balancing and libido-loving ingredients, such as maca powder. Not as thick and creamy as my Supremo Breakfast Smoothie (page 64) but a bit sweeter, which sometimes I just love first thing in the morning.

Add all the ingredients to a blender and blitz until smooth. Pour into a glass and enjoy.

serves 1

½ frozen banana
1 teaspoon maca powder
1 teaspoon camu camu powder
30g spinach
1 teaspoon cacao powder
50g blueberries
30g gluten-free rolled oats

V

serves 2

250ml nut milk, such as almond
60g spinach
200g blueberries
1 kiwi, peeled
3–4 mint leaves
a few ice cubes

V

serves 1

250ml water
½ frozen banana, roughly
   chopped
50g blueberries
30g spinach
1 tablespoon nut butter, such as
   almond
20g vanilla protein powder
a handful of ice cubes
1 teaspoon chia seeds (optional)

V

serves 1

250ml coconut milk
6–8 strawberries
1 teaspoon flaxseeds
juice of ½ lime
2 tablespoons coconut yogurt
2 ice cubes
1 teaspoon maca powder

polar berry

The combination of kiwi, mint and blueberries gives this smoothie an incredibly refreshing feel and taste. You can mix it up by adding hydrating coconut water instead of nut milk.

Pour the nut milk into a blender. Add the spinach, fruit and mint leaves, top with the ice cubes and blend until smooth. Pour into two glasses and enjoy.

the warrior

You've just hit up beast mode in the gym and it's time to replenish your body with this awesome smoothie. With 20g organic plant-based protein and amazing fats to repair your battle-broken body, this is the optimal post-workout smoothie.

Pour half the water into a blender. Add the banana, blueberries, spinach, nut butter and protein powder. Top with the ice and the remaining water and blend until smooth. Serve scattered with the chia seeds, if you wish.

pink flamingo

Ever wake up with some serious holiday blues? Taste your way back to basking in the sun with the tropical Pink Flamingo. Coconut, strawberry and lime – almost a daiquiri.

Pour the coconut milk into a blender and top with the remaining ingredients. Blend until smooth. Pour into a glass and enjoy.

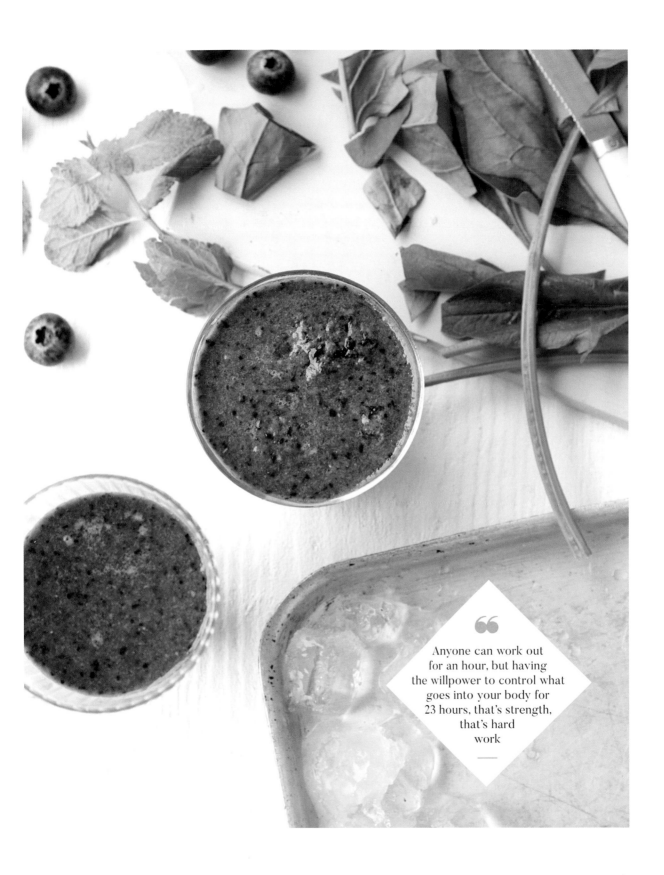

Anyone can work out
for an hour, but having
the willpower to control what
goes into your body for
23 hours, that's strength,
that's hard
work

JUICES

For me, juicing is my way of giving my body that extra helping hand to try to absorb every micronutrient it needs in order to be fabulously flawsome. Organic cold-pressed juices are an amazingly simple way to improve your overall wellbeing. Your body is always welcoming new levels of healthiness that will leave you feeling more glowy, energetic and rejuvenated than ever before.

spring clean

serves 2

2 celery sticks, roughly chopped
1 cucumber, peeled and roughly chopped
juice of 1 lemon
4 mint leaves
a small bunch of coriander
300g pineapple, roughly chopped

Spring-clean your body with this refreshing detox beverage. Cucumber is one of nature's most beneficial anti-inflammatories, aiding digestion and rehydrating the body.

Juice all the ingredients following the instructions on your juicer. It's best to drink the juice immediately to get the maximum benefits of all the nutrients.

hot h2O

serves 2

1 litre water
juice of 1 lemon
juice of 1 lime
2cm piece of fresh ginger, peeled
¼ teaspoon cayenne pepper

I been drinking, I been drinking. According to the media, Queen B (Beyoncé) also loves to dissolve and eliminate toxins and congestion that have formed in any part of her body using this drink. If it's good enough for Bey, pass me the jug.

Mix all the ingredients together in a jug. Pour into two glasses and enjoy.

tip

Juices and smoothies do have a very short shelf life, so it is highly recommended that you consume the juice immediately to reap all the benefits of the vitamins they contain.

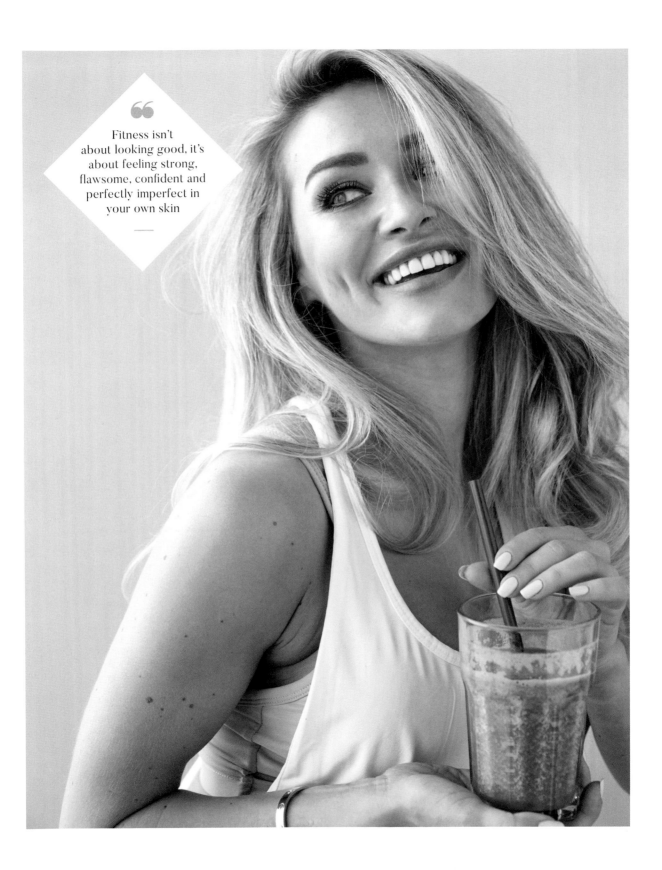

serves 2

2 raw beetroots, scrubbed and
roughly chopped

4 carrots, scrubbed and roughly
chopped

½ cucumber, peeled and roughly
chopped

juice of 1 lemon

¼ teaspoon cayenne pepper

serves 2

½ cucumber, peeled and roughly
chopped

4 celery stalks, chopped

30g kale

30g spinach

1 unwaxed lemon, peeled and
quartered

3cm piece of fresh ginger,
peeled

serves 2

3 carrots, scrubbed and roughly
chopped

¼ lime

1cm piece of fresh ginger, peeled

gimme a beet

The earthiness of beetroots is rather easily disguised by
the sweetness of carrots and the refreshing cucumber juice.
Beetroots or beets, aka blood turnips, are packed with iron
and calcium, which support cleansing by increasing levels of an
antioxidant in the body that is beneficial for liver detoxification.
If you've had too many shots the night before, double the
amount of beets and halve the rest of the ingredients and a shot
of this will get you off the floor.

Juice all the ingredients following the instructions on your juicer. It's
best to drink the juice immediately to get the maximum benefits of all
the nutrients.

emerald isle

If you want to start adding green juices to your lifestyle, this is
a great place to start. A refreshing blend of alkalising greens,
gentle for the digestion and supporting detoxification. Good
health, good luck and happiness, for today and every day.

Juice all the ingredients following the instructions on your juicer. It's
best to drink the juice immediately to get the maximum benefits of all
the nutrients.

vitamin c

To improve your zest for life, fill it with vitamin C.

Juice all the ingredients following the instructions on your juicer. It's
best to drink the juice immediately to get the maximum benefits of all
the nutrients.

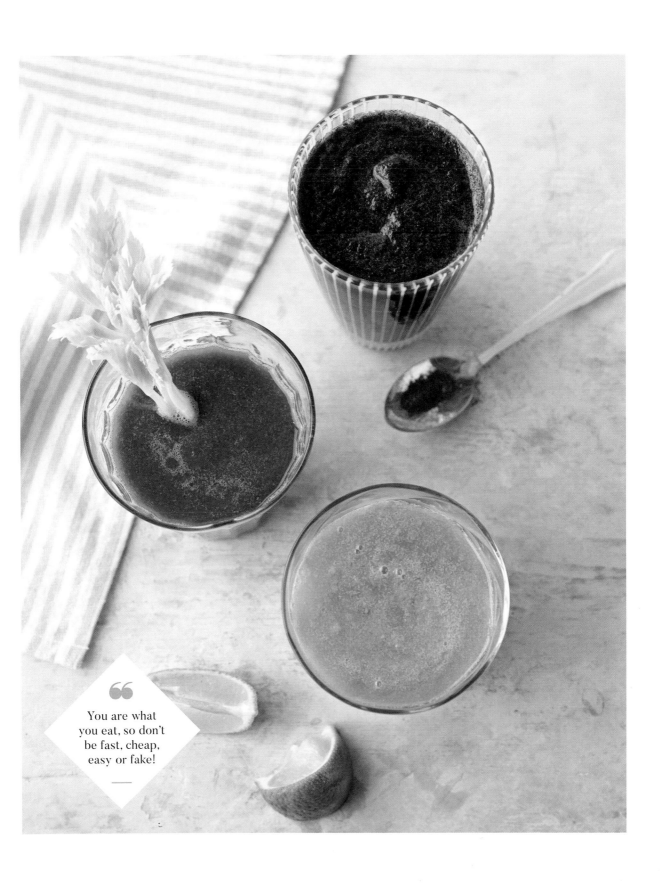

> **"** You are what you eat, so don't be fast, cheap, easy or fake!

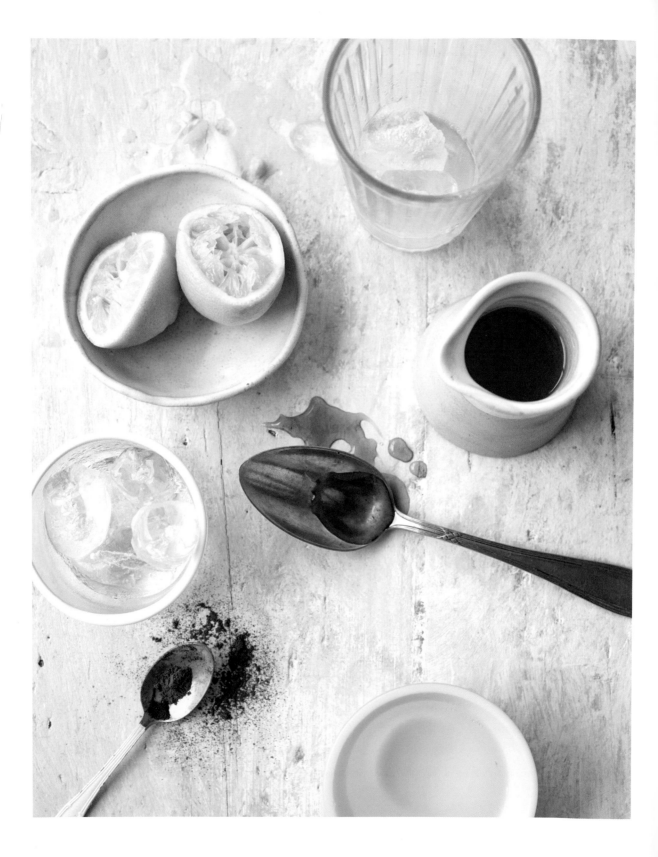

clean green

Chlorophyll helps to boost your immune system and promotes healthy digestion, alongside many other health benefits. It can also taste a bit like pond, but for glowing skin, I'll drink it.

Mix the chlorella powder with the water until dissolved. Sip throughout the day.

serves 1

1 teaspoon chlorella powder
500ml water

first aid

Packed full of greens, including mineral-rich spirulina and chlorella, this drink will maintain the body's natural pH due to its high mineral content. Chlorella is also believed to reduce the chances of getting a hangover – I'll let you decide whether the myth is true or false!

Juice all the ingredients following the instructions on your juicer. It's best to drink the juice immediately to get the maximum benefits of all the nutrients.

serves 2

2 handfuls of spinach
½ cucumber, peeled and roughly
    chopped
juice of 1 lime
½ teaspoon spirulina
½ teaspoon chlorella powder
2cm piece of fresh ginger,
    peeled

zeus juice

For times when you just need that little extra lightning bolt of energy.

Juice all the ingredients following the instructions on your juicer. It's best to drink the juice immediately to get the maximum benefits of all the nutrients.

serves 2

4cm piece of fresh ginger,
    peeled
juice of 1 lemon
2cm piece of fresh turmeric or
    ½ teaspoon ground turmeric
a grinding of black pepper

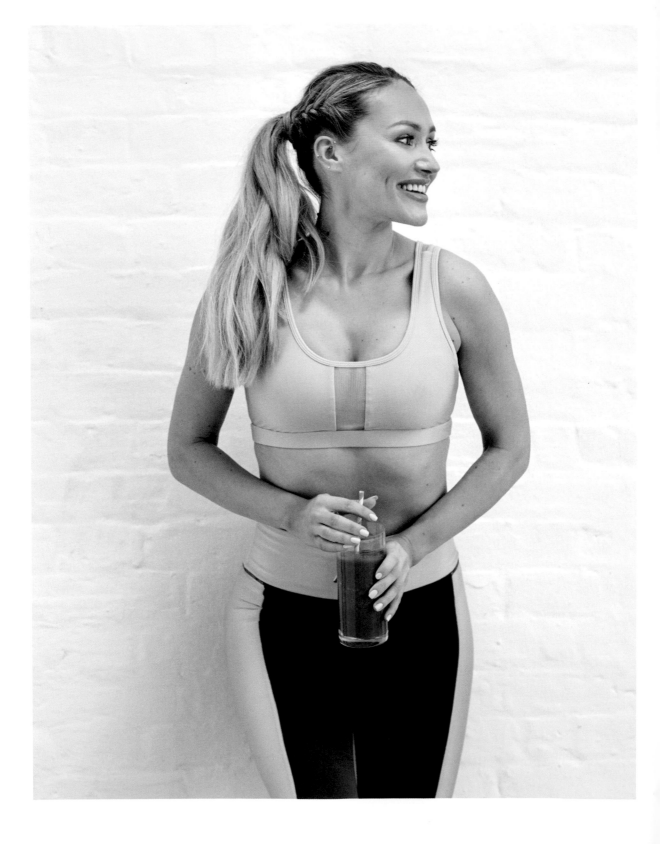

the
workouts

In this section I have provided you with both home and gym workouts, at Beginner and Advanced levels. From 15–45 minutes long, there is a range of fitspirational home workouts for you to do. I recommend doing my workouts 3–4 times a week and getting 30 minutes of activity into your life every day.

If for some reason you are unable to perform these workouts due to medical conditions, I recommend taking advice from your doctor about how you can do alternative exercises to avoid remaining completely sedentary.

Never get discouraged; every single effort you put in is changing your body. You might not always love the workout, but you will always love the results!

my top workout tips

Getting fit and staying fit is a challenge in itself, so how do you stay motivated?

Remind yourself, it's never too late to work towards being a healthier, fitter version of you. Getting the motivation to exercise is all in your head; I work out because I love my body, not because I hate it.

Everyone can have a hard time making exercise part of their daily routine, and I have no doubt that if you have kids it can feel even more impossible to create the time, but there are so many health benefits that come from exercising. One hour is just 4 per cent of your day, so 30 minutes is only 2 per cent – that's not even a full episode on Netflix! If you have time to Netflix and chill, you can roll out a mat and try one of my home workout routines. Get out of your comfort zone – yes, it may be a comfortable place but, hey, nothing is going to change there. Become an early bird with me.

It's true what they say, a goal without a plan is just a wish. Perhaps I'm your motivational fairy, so imagine I am sprinkling some motivational dust on you and now you can go and make your wishes come true.

Try to follow an effective planned workout routine. I like to schedule my workouts into my days. I make them part of my everyday life, so I know that when I wake up first thing in the morning I am hitting the gym or rolling out the yoga mat to do a workout. I know that if I leave my workout until the evening there is only a 50/50 chance I'm going to make it.

Mondays are always a great day to start – everyone is feeling super motivated, getting to the gym with high hopes of powering through a week of epic workouts. But the hustle and bustle of a packed gym on a Monday can also be offputting, so I like to ease into my workouts at the weekend, when I know I can set aside plenty of time and the gym will be much quieter.

Before you hit the gym, there are a few things you might want to consider, to get you motivated and keep you going.

◆ **HYDRATION:** Proper hydration before, during and after your workout is key to your performance. Building up a sweat is great but it also results in a loss of fluid from your body. As you dehydrate your performance levels drop, so drinking water during exercise is essential if you want to get the most out of your workout.

◆ **SLEEP:** Getting quality sleep is just as important as your workout routine and good nutrition. If getting lean and toned is your primary goal, getting 8 hours of sleep a night is the base on which a healthy body and mind function.

◆ **GIVE YOURSELF A REST DAY:** This is just as important as working out. In order to repair and strengthen your body you must give it adequate rest or you will not benefit from all the hard work you are putting in. If you decide not to have a rest day you are putting yourself at greater risk of injury. Take these workout-free days to reflect on how much you have achieved and be grateful for your body.

◆ **MUSIC:** Have a killer playlist ready to go. If I leave my headphones at home, chances are I'm going back to get them. Having a good playlist always gets me motivated and in the zone. The rhythm of music can aid self-paced workouts like running and weight-lifting, too. I don't necessarily listen to the latest songs, but upbeat, fast-paced dance music always keeps me going. Think 90s club anthems, high-energy, mood-boosting songs to power you through your workout.

◆ **CLOTHING:** Do gym clothes really affect your workouts? I think they do. There is nothing worse than wearing leggings that you have to keep yanking up or worrying that they will become see-through when you squat. Bouncing boobs are another no-no when it comes to running and high-intensity routines. Being

supported, dry and comfortable is essential when it comes to exercising, and we all want to look fashionably fit, so invest in brands that really specialise in activewear.

◆ **GET INSPIRED:** The fact that you are not where you want to be should be motivation enough. We all stand in front of the mirror and self-hate, but that has to stop – negative thoughts are guaranteed to bring you down. We are not perfect, and we don't have to be, but choosing to be the best version of yourself and being grateful for your body is a good step towards loving yourself.

◆ **TAKE BEFORE AND AFTER PICTURES:** We all love to see a good transformation on social media, so why not do one of yourself? Begin by taking a before picture on Day 1 and once you start exercising, take a new set of after pictures every week. Give it a few months for the changes to really show, then compare your photos in a collage. Remember, nobody is built like you, you design yourself.

◆ **CALL IN THE PROS:** Consider working with a personal trainer, if not in every session, then maybe just every once in a while. I do this myself and having that one-to-one time with an expert encourages you to make it to that workout and really push yourself hard. Even though I am a fully qualified trainer, I enjoy learning new skills and making sure my form is always on point. A personal trainer will be able to teach you the proper form for each exercise, so if you find heading to the weights room a little daunting, learning how to properly perform exercises won't only boost your confidence but reduce the risk of injury, too.

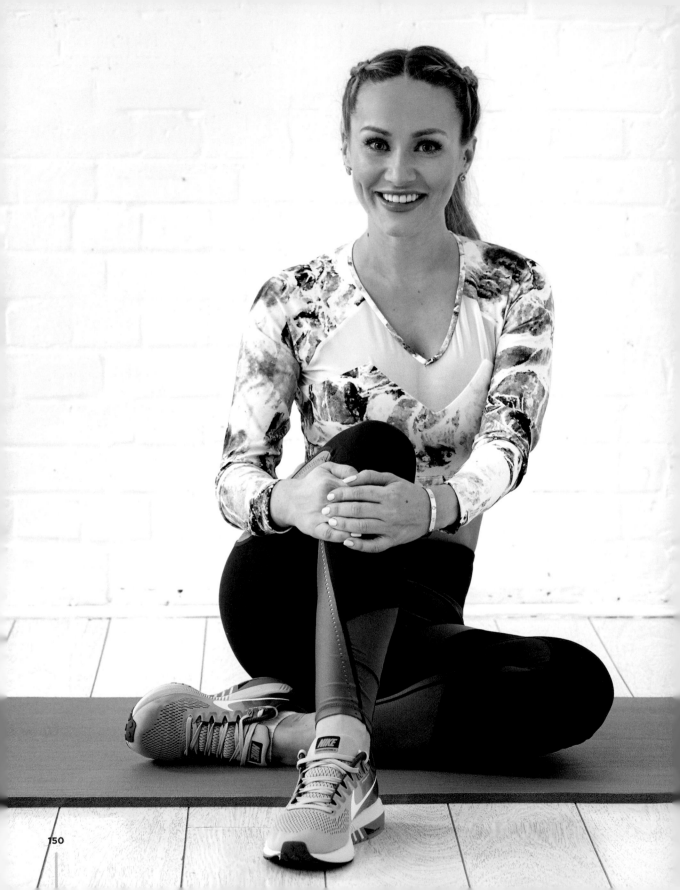

CHALLENGE YOURSELF

If your workout is not challenging you it sure as hell isn't going to change you. Keep challenging yourself throughout your workouts and you will keep progressing. When you bring that effort, that hunger for change, every single day that's when transformations happen. Have you hit your goal? Then set a new one, that's how change continues to occur.

WEAR A FITNESS TRACKER: Does it even count if I haven't tracked it? What motivates me to work out most is my fitness tracker. Monitoring my movement throughout the day and my workouts reminds me to keep moving.

GOALS

Goals are individual, not universal. Just because someone can lift heavier weights, work out more or lose weight quicker, doesn't mean that your effort isn't valid. You work hard for you, this is your lifestyle and your own goals. Set a goal that is so meaningful it creates a positive, powerful drive inside you, a drive to become better and stronger. Progress will come. It's time to set some goals. Please make them realistic. Aiming to look like a *Sports Illustrated* model in a week? Time to get off your unicorn.

YOUR GOALS NEED TO BE:

Specific
Measurable
Attainable
Relevant
Timed
Evaluative
Revisable

Write it down, put it on a Post-it on your mirror so you can see it every day. Set an alarm on your phone to remind yourself, make a moodboard of inspirational quotes, images or workout routines, whatever inspires you to maintain the focus and discipline throughout your process. No matter how many mistakes you make or how slow you are going, remember you are still moving forward, better than yesterday and way ahead of everyone who isn't trying.

At the end of the day, do it for you, because making yourself proud is one of the best feelings in the world.

stretching

> **"**
> A good full-body stretching routine is key to getting stronger and expanding your range of motion
> —

Stretching is important for a number of different reasons – to reduce muscle fatigue, enhance flexibility and sports performance, lessen the risk of injury, improve posture and prevent muscle soreness. When exercising, your muscles shorten from the constant contractions you are performing, so stretching returns them to their original length.

Coming from an athletic background, I have been trained to do a small warm-up and plenty of dynamic stretching before each workout. I find warming up the body with 8 minutes of steady state cardio and lighter moves of my upcoming workout enough for my body to adjust to the demands of the exercises I will be performing. However, stretching before your workout when not fully warmed up can actually cause the muscles to tighten, resulting in a greater risk of injury, so I recommend stretching after a workout, because then your muscles are already warmed up and full of blood.

I take 10–15 minutes to stretch out my muscles after working out, because stretching after exercise is a great feel-good way to finish up. A good full-body stretching routine is key to getting stronger and expanding your range of motion. The following drills will help you move better by increasing your flexibility. Think about slow control and breathing deeply into each movement.

Hold each stretch for 15–30 seconds

CHILD'S POSE
(left + right stretch)

1. Perform Child's Pose following the instructions on page 30.
2. Keeping your legs and pelvis aligned, pull your torso over to your left side, keeping your arms and head in the same position.
3. Repeat on the opposite side.

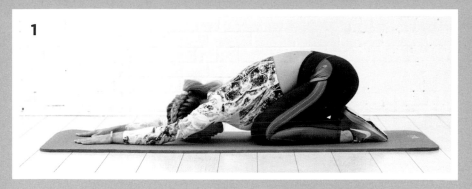

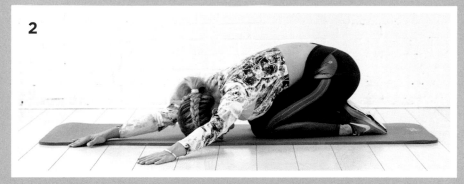

KNEELING GROIN STRETCH
(left + right stretch)

1. Stand with your feet shoulder-width apart and take a large step forward with your right leg. Allow your left knee to come down to touch the floor. Your left shin and the top of your left foot should be flat against the mat.
2. Push your pelvis forward and hold, keeping your back straight. Release and repeat on the opposite side.

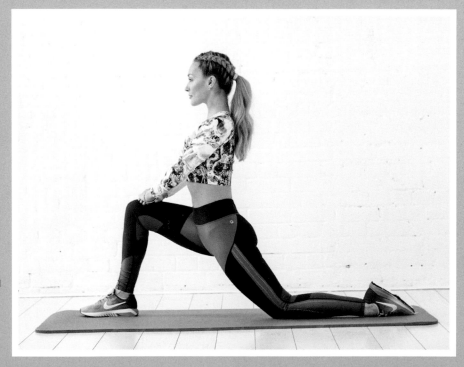

PIGEON POSE
(left + right)

1. Start on your hands and knees. Bring your right leg forward and cross below your body. Slide your left leg back, keeping your knee to the ground.
2. While exhaling, walk your hands forward and lower your upper body to the floor. Hold for 15–20 seconds.
3. Push back through your hands and slowly release.
4. Repeat on the opposite side.

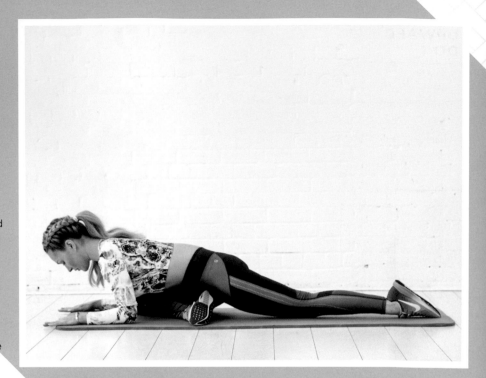

LOW LUNGE
(left + right)

1. Start in Downward Dog (page 155). Exhale, step your right foot forward. Lower yourself onto your left knee.
2. While inhaling, bring yourself upright with your spine straight.
3. Exhale and bring your hands back to the floor. Slightly raise your left knee to complete the stretch.
4. Repeat on the opposite side.

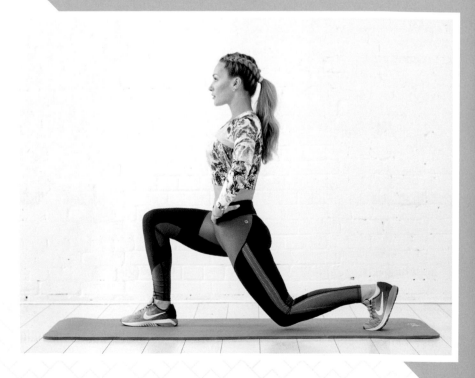

UPWARD DOG

1. Start lying face-down on the floor. Bend your arms and bring your hands face-down on the floor just above parallel to your waist.
2. Inhale, press your hands firmly into the floor. Straighten your arms and lift your back, waist and tops of your legs a few inches off the floor.
3. Keep your bum firm but not tensed. Tip your head back slightly and hold for 30 seconds.

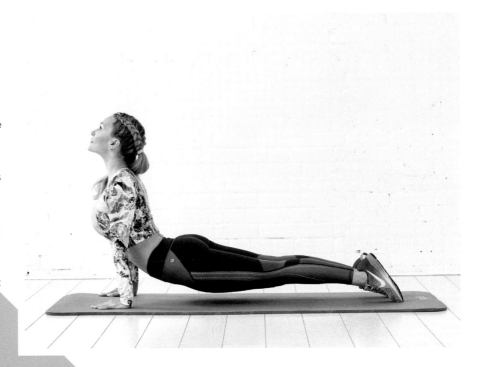

DOWNWARD DOG

1. Start on your hands and knees. Exhale and push your pelvis towards the ceiling. Slowly begin to straighten your legs.
2. Keep your arms extended and push away from the floor, lifting through your pelvis. Heels should be slightly raised. Hold for 15–20 seconds.
3. To release, exhale and bend through your knees, bringing yourself back to the starting position.

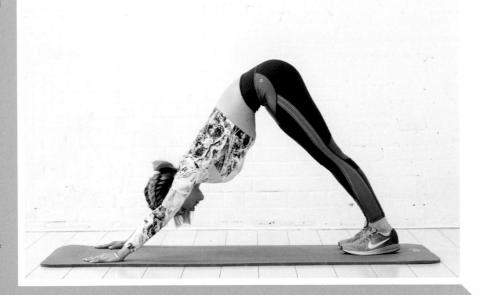

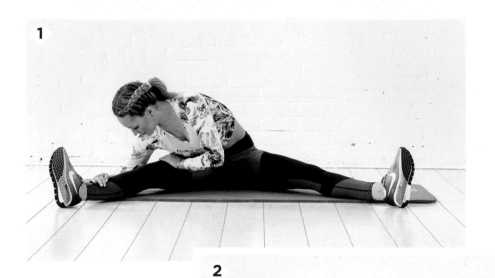

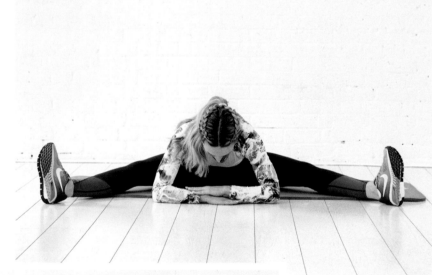

HEAD TO KNEE
(right, centre, left)

1. Start by sitting on the floor with your legs stretched out open in front of you. Bring your torso over to your right knee and rest your arms on your right leg. Lower your head and sternum and hold for 1 minute, release and return to the starting position.

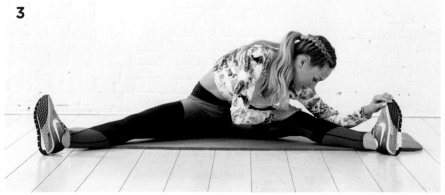

2. Cross your arms and lower your head, sternum and torso straight in front of you pushing into the stretch. Hold for 1 minute and release, returning to the starting position.

3. Repeat step 1 on your left side.

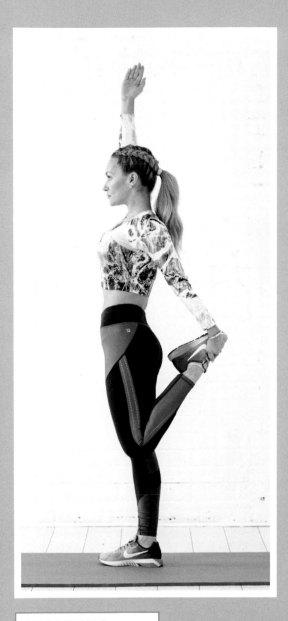

REACH BACK
CHEST STRETCH

1. Start in a standing position, with your feet just under shoulder-width apart.
2. Bring your arms back behind your back and clasp your hands together. While keeping your arms straight, pull them backwards and push your sternum forwards and slightly towards the ceiling. Hold, release and repeat.

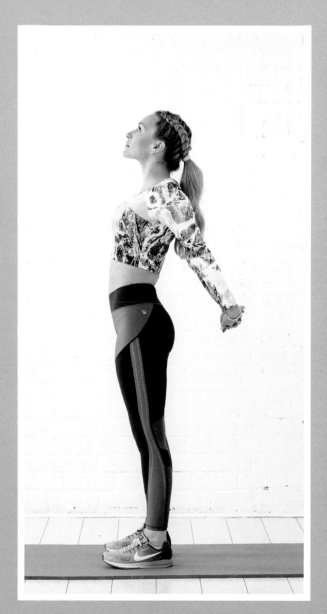

STANDING
QUAD STRETCH
(left + right)

1. Start standing with your feet together. Bend your left knee and bring your left ankle towards your bum. Clasp your ankle with your left hand, use your right hand to keep balance.
2. Push your left hip slightly forward so that you can begin to feel the stretch. Keep your knees together. Hold for 30 seconds and repeat on the opposite side.

LATERAL NECK STRETCH

1. Stand with your feet shoulder-width apart. Bring your right arm over the top of your head and rest your palm against the left hand side of your head. Keep your left arm out straight.
2. Generating resistance with your neck, push your right hand against your face so that you can feel the stretch. Hold this position and repeat on the opposite side.

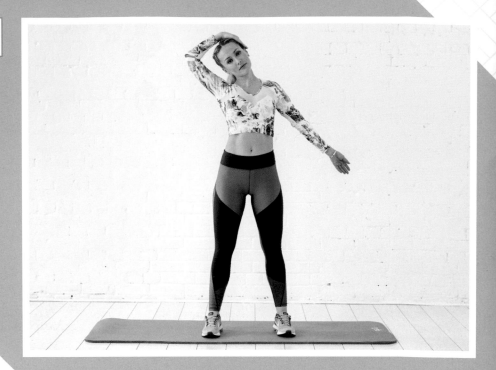

ARM CROSSOVER SHOULDER STRETCH

1. Stand with your feet shoulder-width apart. Bring your right arm across your body to your left hand side, keeping it straight at all times. Fold your left arm over your right arm and pull against your right arm. Hold.
2. Repeat on the opposite side.

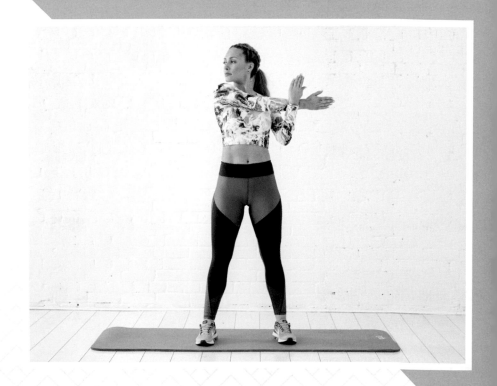

FORWARD FOLD HOLD

1. Stand with your feet slightly narrower than shoulder-width apart.
2. Exhale and hinge forward from your hips. You might need to bend your knees a little to bring your palms around your ankles.
3. Continue to bend and if possible press your forehead against your knees. Hold for 10–15 seconds.
4. Inhale as you release and bend further from the knees if necessary.

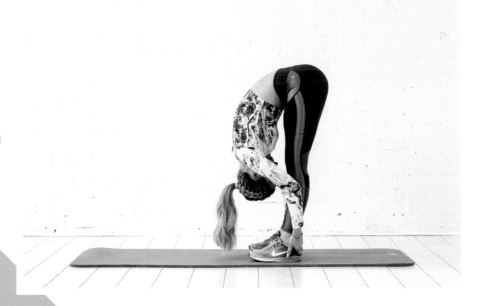

UPPER BACK STRETCH

1. Stand with your feet shoulder-width apart. Clasp your hands together in front of you, keep your arms straight and raise them to shoulder height.
2. Keep your torso tall and push the stretch through your upper back. Hold and repeat.

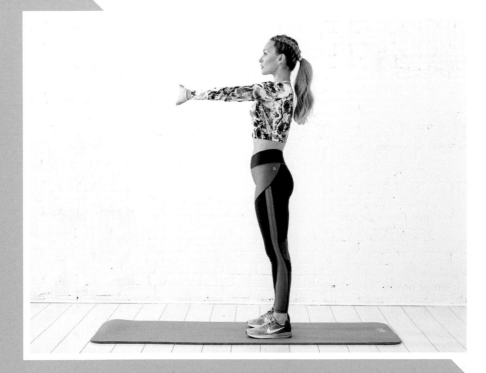

> **You've got this!! Ready? Let's go.**

home workouts

ZERO EQUIPMENT NEEDED
ZERO EXCUSES

My home workout plan requires minimal-to-no equipment and is exactly what you need to get in shape in the comfort of your own home. Each workout will challenge you from different angles and use a full range of motions, embrace your core and keep your form controlled and strong. As you progress, remember to increase the intensity of your workouts.

Let's start by building overall strength with my circuit-style time- and rep-based exercises. Use my warm-ups first to prepare for all the following exercises (pages 164–167).

Remember to keep track of how many reps of each exercise you're able to do, increasing the number from week to week. This should help you to stay motivated and push your limits to improve as much as you can. Start your week strong, finish your week stronger!

Make sure that you take a few minutes before each workout to warm up and do some dynamic stretching. Post-workout, do my full body stretching routine on pages 153–159.

upper body

SET 1

- **PLANK WALKS (p.168)**
  x 30 seconds

- **TRICEP DIPS (p.182)**
  x 30 seconds

- **WALK OUT –
  BURPEE JUMPS (p.176)**
  x 30 seconds

- **PLANK SAWS (p.169)**
  x 30 seconds

- **PLANK WALKS (p.168)**
  x 30 seconds

- **TRICEP DIPS (p.182)**
  30 seconds

- **WALK OUT –
  BURPEE JUMPS (p.176)**
  x 30 seconds

- **PLANK SAWS (p.169)**
  x 30 seconds

Rest 1 minute

SET 2

- **SUPERMAN (p.189)**
  x 30 seconds

- **BIRD DOG RIGHT (p.175)**
  x 30 seconds

- **BIRD DOG LEFT (p.175)**
  30 seconds

- **SIDE PLANK RIGHT (p.170)**
  x 30 seconds

- **SIDE PLANK LEFT (p.170)**
  x 30 seconds

- **PLANK WALKS (p.168)**
  x 30 seconds

- **MOUNTAIN CLIMBERS (p.173)**
  x 30 seconds

- **SUPERMAN (p.189)**
  x 30 seconds

- **BIRD DOG RIGHT (p.175)**
  x 30 seconds

- **BIRD DOG LEFT (p.175)**
  x 30 seconds

- **SIDE PLANK RIGHT (p.170)**
  x 30 seconds

- **SIDE PLANK LEFT (p.170)**
  x 30 seconds

- **PLANK WALKS (p.168)**
  x 30 seconds

Rest 1 minute

SET 3

- **MOUNTAIN CLIMBERS (p.173)**
  x 30 seconds

- **BURPEE HOPS (p.175)**
  x 30 seconds

Rest 30 seconds

- **MOUNTAIN CLIMBERS (p.173)**
  x 30 seconds

- **BURPEE HOPS (p.175)**
  x 30 seconds

Rest 30 seconds

- **MOUNTAIN CLIMBERS
  (p.173)** x 30 seconds

- **BURPEE HOPS (p.173)**
  x 30 seconds

Rest 30 seconds

lower body

WARM-UP x 2

- **HIGH KNEE MARCH (p.165)** x 20

- **REVERSE LUNGES (p.179)** x 10

- **KNEE HUGS (p.182)** x 10

- **WALK OUTS (p.167)** x 10

- **HIP LIFTS (p.177)** x 10

- **FORWARD LUNGES (p.178)** x 10

Rest 30 seconds

SET 1 x 2

- **WALKING LUNGES (p.195)** x 30

- **V UPS (p.188)** x 15

- **BURPEES (p.175)** x 12

Rest 30 seconds

SET 2 x 2

- **LATERAL LUNGES (p.178)** x 30

- **PLANK TOE TAPS (p.170)** x 12

Rest 30 seconds

SET 3 x 2

- **SPLIT JUMPS (p.181)** x 30

- **PLANK REACHES (p.173)** x 12

Rest 30 seconds

SET 4 x 2

- **BODYWEIGHT SQUATS
  (p.185)** x 30

TRiCEP DIPS (p.182) x 15

bums & tums

- Working with a full range of movement, get ready to really challenge your core and glutes.

- Be precise and keep your form strong.

Perform each movement for 1 minute (little–no rest).

- ♦ BIRD DOGS (p.175)

- ♦ BOTTOM UP SQUATS (p.184)

- ♦ SINGLE-LEG HIP RAISES (p.188)

Perform each movement for 40 seconds with 20 seconds rest between each exercise.

- ♦ PLANK SAWS (p.169)

- ♦ CRUNCH TOE TOUCHES (p.189)

- ♦ SIDE PLANK RIGHT/LEFT (p.170)

- ♦ PLANK TOE TAPS (p.170)

Perform each movement for 1 minute (little–no rest).

- ♦ BODYWEIGHT SQUATS (p.185)

- ♦ CROSS BACK LUNGES (p.189)

- ♦ FORWARD LUNGES (p.178)

Perform each movement for 40 seconds with 20 seconds rest between each exercise.

- ♦ LEG RAISES (p.186)

- ♦ PLANK LEG LIFTS (p.169)

- ♦ LEG RAISES (p.186)

- ♦ PLANK SAWS (p.169)

- ♦ LEG RAISES (p.186)

- ♦ PLANK (p.168)

Perform each movement for 1 minute (little–no rest).

- ♦ HIP LIFTS (p.177)

- ♦ SIDE-LEG LIFTS LEFT/ RIGHT (p.180)

- ♦ SUMO SQUATS (p.183)

Perform each movement for 40 seconds with 20 seconds rest between each exercise.

- ♦ ALTERNATING LEG RAISES (p.186)

- ♦ PLANK TOE TAPS (p.170)

- ♦ CRUNCH TOE TOUCHES (p.189)

- ♦ PLANK SHOULDER TAPS (p.172)

8-minute abs workout

Try to add my 8-minute abs workout to the end of either your home or gym workouts for the ultimate burn!

Traditional core exercises, such as crunches or bicycles, are great for sculpting your upper abdominals and obliques. But are they really working your full core? No, not even close. Imagine all that painful crunching is barely touching those pesky lower abs, and, let's be honest, the lower abs are more often than not a trouble spot for us all. So how do we banish the muffin?

Are you short on time? Missed the gym or just want a quick at-home abs blast? Don't worry, just try this 8-minute ab burner or add it to the end of any workout.

Perform each movement for 1 minute and rest for 20 seconds between exercises.

- ♦ ALTERNATING LEG RAISES (p.186)

- ♦ PLANK TOE TAPS (p.170)

- ♦ CRUNCH TOE TOUCHES (p.189)

- ♦ SCISSOR CRUNCHES (p.191)

- ♦ PLANK SAWS (p.169)

- ♦ FLUTTER KICKS (p.190)

- ♦ PLANK DROPS (p.172)

- ♦ MOUNTAIN CLIMBERS (p.173)

full body

WARM-UP
Repeat each move for
30 seconds with no rest
in between each exercise.

- ♦ **HIGH KNEE MARCH (p.165)**
- ♦ **WALK OUTS (p.167)**
- ♦ **HIP OPENERS (p.164)**
- ♦ **DYNAMIC QUAD STRETCH (p.166)**
- ♦ **HIGH KNEE MARCH (p.165)**
- ♦ **WALK OUTS (p.167)**
- ♦ **DYNAMIC HAMSTRING STRETCH (p.164)**

SET 1
Repeat each move for
30 seconds with no rest
in between each exercise.

- ♦ **REVERSE LUNGES (p.179)**
- ♦ **PLANK WALKS (p.168)**
- ♦ **BODYWEIGHT SQUATS (p.185)**
- ♦ **WALK OUT – BURPEE JUMPS (p.176)**
- ♦ **MOUNTAIN CLIMBERS (p.173)**

Rest 30 seconds

SET 2
Repeat each move for
30 seconds with no rest in
between each exercise.

- ♦ **REVERSE LUNGES (p.179)**
- ♦ **PLANK WALKS (p.168)**
- ♦ **PLANK LEG LIFTS (p.169)**
- ♦ **BODYWEIGHT SQUATS (p.185)**
- ♦ **WALK OUT – BURPEE JUMPS (p.176)**
- ♦ **BURPEES (p.174)**

Rest 1 minute

SET 3
CORE

Repeat each move from the
previous sets for
50 seconds with no rest
in between each exercise.

high intensity

WARM-UP x 2

- ♦ **WALK OUTS (p.167)** x 10
- ♦ **REVERSE LUNGE STRETCH (p.180)** x 10
- ♦ **HIGH KNEE MARCH (p.165)** x 20

SET 1

- ♦ **SPLIT JUMPS (p.181)** x 10
- ♦ **SQUAT JUMPS (p.183)** x 10
- ♦ **BURPEES (p.174)** x 10

Rest 10 seconds

SET 2

As Set 1 repeating each exercise
8 times.

SET 3 x 2

As Set 1 repeating each exercise
6 times.

SET 4

As Set 1 repeating each exercise
4 times.

SET 5

As Set 1 repeating each exercise
2 times.

COOL DOWN (pages 213–217)

warm-up

HIP OPENERS

1. Start the move standing tall with your feet shoulder-width apart.
2. Step out to the right hand side whilst keeping your feet and torso facing forwards. Bend your right knee and lower your torso so that your arms are relaxed and touching the floor.
3. Hold and repeat on the opposite side.

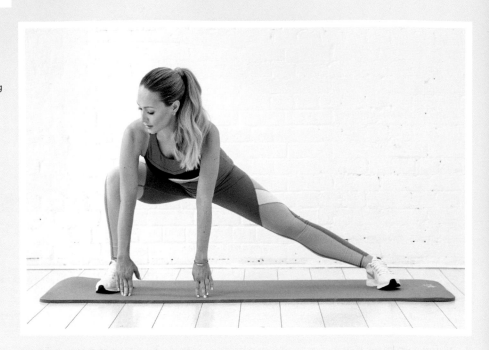

DYNAMIC HAMSTRING STRETCH

1. Start the move standing tall with your feet shoulder-width apart. Put your hands on your waist and step forward with your right leg.
2. Bend your right knee and push into the stretch.
3. Repeat on the opposite leg and continue the movement until you have completed 10 stretches on each side.

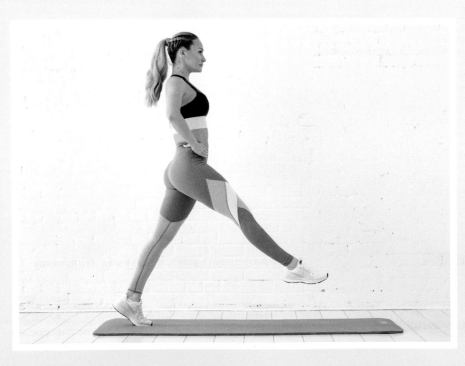

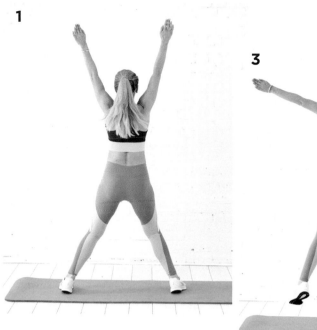

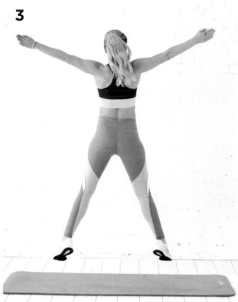

STAR JUMPS

1. Stand with knees slightly bent and feet shoulder-width apart. Your arms should be slightly bent at your sides.
2. Bend your knees to get into a squat position and jump as high as you can. Extend your legs and arms fully out to your sides at the same time in mid-air to form a star shape with your body. Your arms should point upward at a 45-degree angle away from your head.

3. Squat and push off again to perform a second star jump. This exercise can be done repeatedly. By pulling your limbs inward on the descent, you prepare yourself for successive jumps.

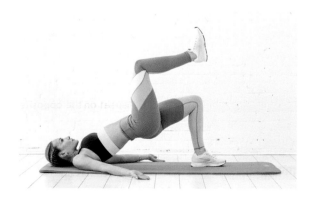

HIGH KNEE MARCH

1. Start by lying on your back with your shoulders flat against the floor. Bend both knees and pull your feet towards your bottom.
2. Pushing through your legs, raise your hips towards the ceiling, with your shoulders pressed firmly into the ground and arms flat against the floor. Raise your right leg keeping your knee bent.
3. Return your leg to the floor and repeat on the opposite leg. Repeat for 10 stretches on each side.

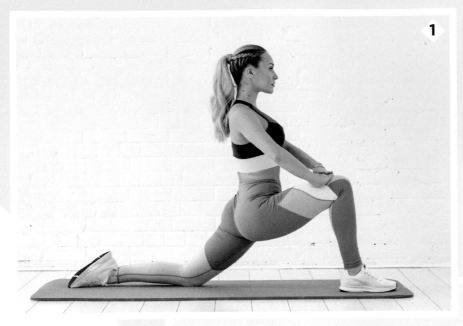

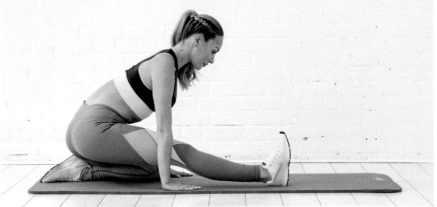

DYNAMIC QUAD STRETCH

1. Start the move by kneeling with your torso up straight.
2. Bring your right leg forward so that your right foot is flat on the ground. Stretch your left leg out behind you and ensure that your left shin keeps contact with the floor and the top of your left foot is facing down.
3. Pull yourself back from this position so that your right leg is straight out in front of you with the foot flexed and your bottom is resting on your left heel.
   Repeat on the opposite leg and continue until you have completed 10 stretches on each side.

WALK OUTS

1. Bend at the hips and plant your hands on the floor, shoulder-width apart, a couple of inches in front of your feet.
2. Walk your hands forwards until your body is in a push-up/plank position.
3. Do one push up. Walk your hands back to the starting position.

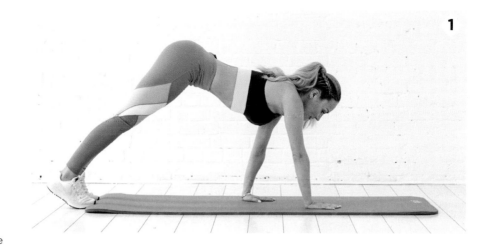

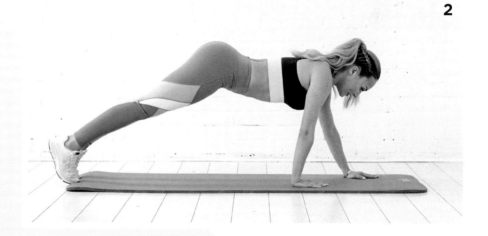

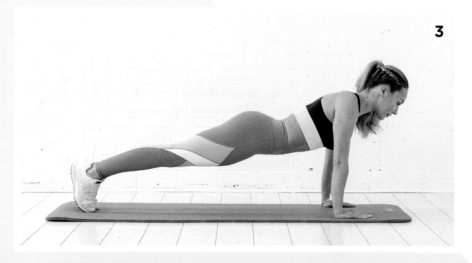

exercises

PLANK

1. Start by lying on the floor. Place your forearms on the mat parallel to each other, a few inches apart.
2. Raise your torso, while keeping your core tight and push up onto your toes. Keep your bum slightly raised and hold the position for 15–20 seconds. Straight arm plank can be used as another option.

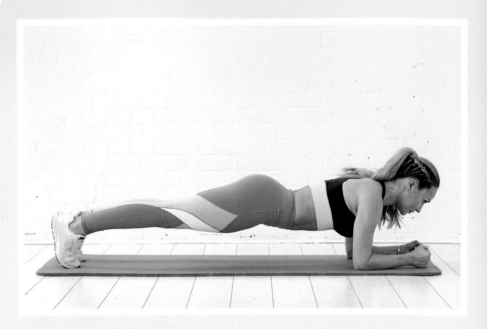

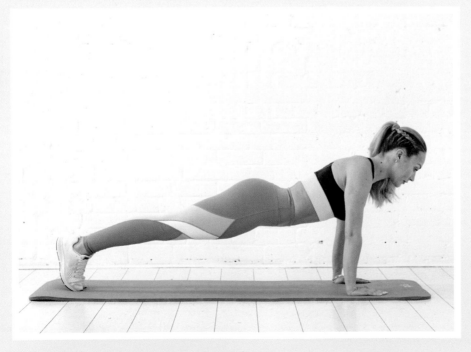

PLANK WALKS

1. Start in a prone plank position, resting on your forearms with your body forming a straight line from shoulders to feet (see above).
2. Push up from the ground, one arm at a time, into the elevated press-up position, all while maintaining your rigid plank form.
3. Repeat.

PLANK LEG LIFTS

1. Start in a plank position with your weight resting on your forearms and toes, elbows directly beneath your shoulders.
2. Brace your core and lift one foot off the floor. Switch legs to complete the rep.

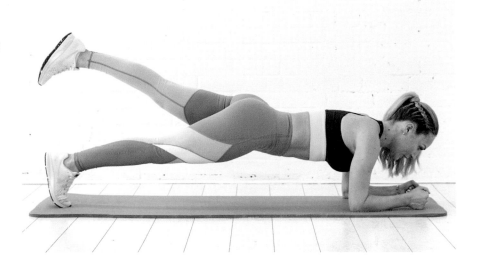

1

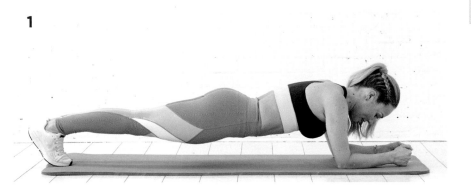

2

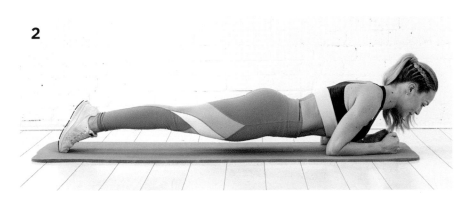

PLANK SAWS

1. Start in a push-up position, bending your elbows 90 degrees and resting your weight on your forearms. Your elbows should be directly beneath your shoulders, and your body should form a straight line from your head to your feet. Squeeze your glutes and tighten your core.
2. Then, push your body backward with your forearms as far as you can. Pull yourself back to the starting position and repeat.

PLANK TOE TAPS

1. Lie face down on the ground and move into a bent arm plank position with your forearms touching the floor. Keep your bum slightly raised and your core tight.
2. Lift your left leg and bring out to the side, tapping your foot to the floor and then reverting back to the original position.
3. Repeat on the opposite side and continue for the desired number of reps.

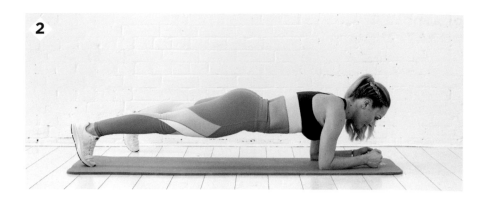

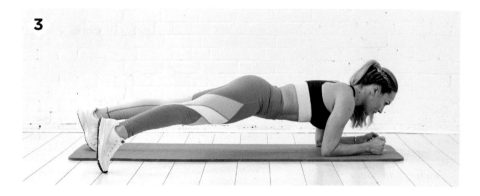

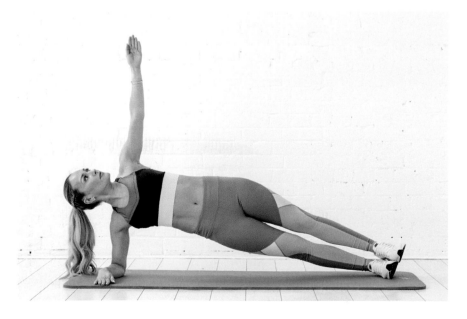

SIDE PLANK

1. Lie on your right side with your legs straight.
2. Prop yourself up with your right forearm so your body forms a diagonal line.
3. Raise your left arm to the ceiling, brace your abs and hold the position for 60 seconds. Be sure your hips and knees stay off the floor.
4. Repeat on the opposite side.

PLANK ROTATIONAL REACH

1. Lie on your left side with your knees straight. Prop your upper body up on your left arm. Brace your abs as if you were about to be punched in the gut.

2. Raise your hips until your body forms a straight line from your ankles to your shoulders. Now raise your right arm straight above you so that it's perpendicular to the floor.

3. Reach under and behind your torso with your right hand, and then lift your arm back up to the starting position.

4. Repeat on the opposite side.

1

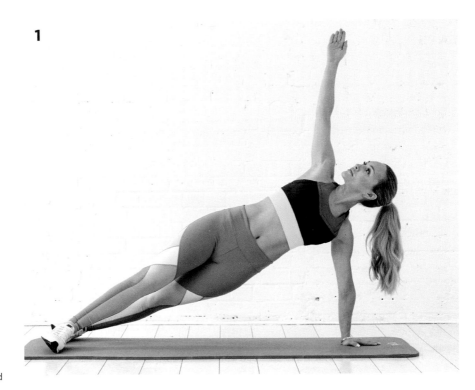

2

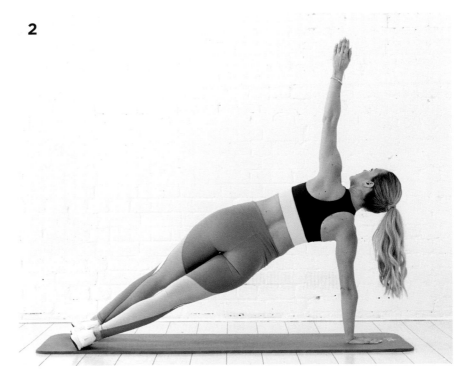

PLANK SHOULDER TAPS

1. Start by lying on the floor face-down and move into a straight arm plank position. Keep your bum slightly raised and your core tight.
2. Raise your right hand to your left shoulder and return to the starting position.
3. Repeat on the opposite side and ensure that your body does not rotate or twist as you complete the move.

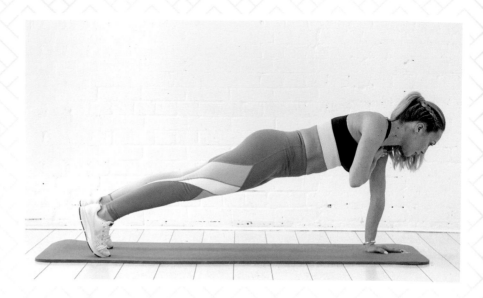

PLANK DROPS

1. Start in plank position (page 168).
2. Rotate at the waist and touch your right hip to the ground.
3. Rotate back up and then to the left and touch your left hip to the ground.
4. Alternate back and forth to complete the repetition.

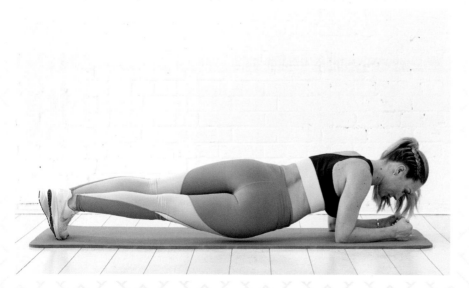

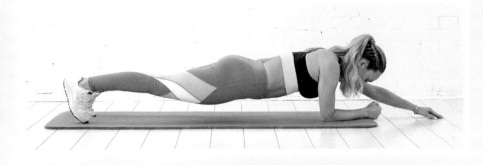

PLANK REACHES

1. Lie face down on the ground and move into forearm plank.
2. Reach your left arm out in front of you.
3. Return to your start position and repeat on the opposite side.

MOUNTAIN CLIMBERS

1. Start in a push-up position with your arms straight and your body in a straight line from your head to your ankles.
2. Without changing the posture of your lower back, raise your right knee towards your chest.
3. Pause, return to the starting position and repeat with your left leg.

1

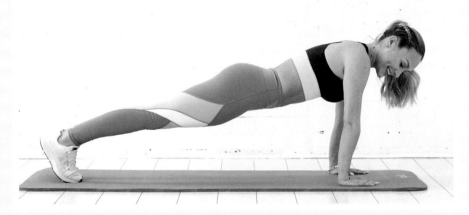

2

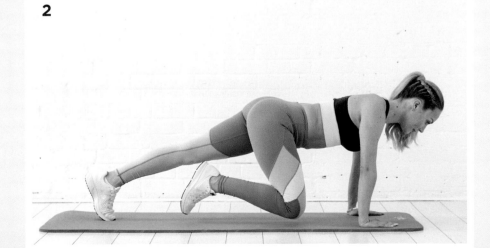

BURPEES

1. Stand with your feet shoulder-width apart, your weight in your heels, and your arms at your sides.
2. Push your hips back, bend your knees, and lower your body into a squat.
3. Place your hands on the floor directly in front of, and just inside, your feet. Shift your weight onto them.
4. Jump your feet back to softly land on the balls of your feet in a plank position. Your body should form a straight line from your head to heels.
5. Jump your feet back so that they land just outside of your hands.
6. Jump explosively into the air.
7. Land and immediately lower yourself back into a squat for your next rep.

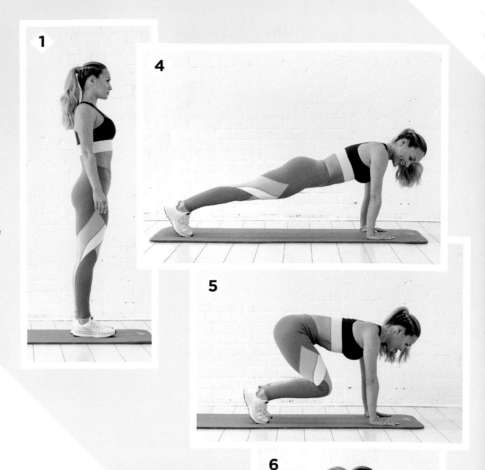

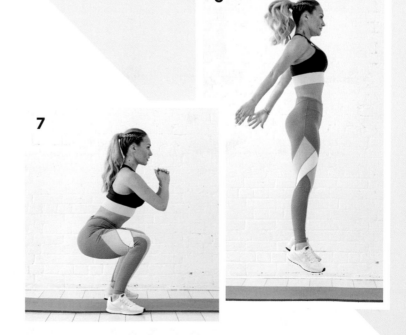

BURPEE HOPS

1. Stand with your feet hip width apart, then squat down and place your hands on the ground in front of you.
2. Jump your legs back into plank position.
3. Jump legs back in between your hands and drive upwards, raising your right knee to the ceiling and pushing through your left leg.
4. Repeat the move on the opposite side.

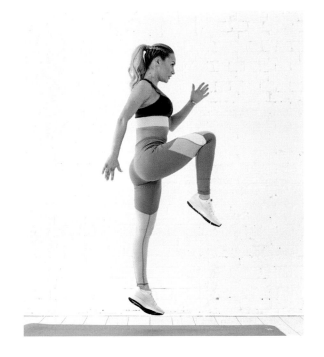

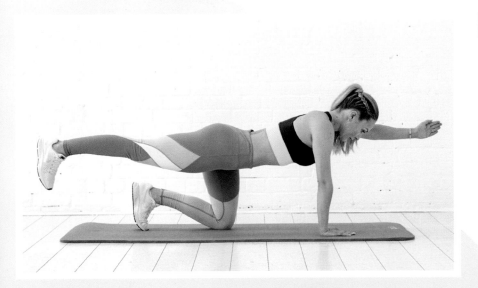

BIRD DOG

1. Start on all fours and tighten your abdominal muscles while keeping your spine and neck in a neutral position.
2. Slowly extend your right leg behind you while reaching your left arm forward. Keep your hips and shoulders square and make sure your lower back doesn't arch.
3. Slowly return to the starting position and repeat the movement on the opposite side.

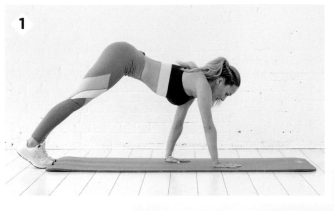

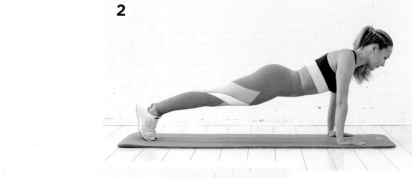

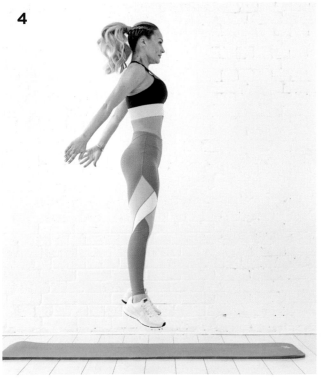

WALK OUT
- BURPEE JUMP

1. Bend at the hips and plant your hands on the floor, shoulder-width apart, a couple of inches in front of your feet.
2. Walk your hands forward until your body is in a push-up/plank position.
3. Do one push up.
4. Jump your feet back to your hands, and from this crouched position jump up. Jump as high up as you can. This completes one rep.
5. Return to your starting position and repeat.

HIP LIFTS

1. Lie on your back with your knees bent and your feet flat on the floor.
2. Place your arms out to your sides at a 45-degree angle.
3. Engage your core and squeeze your glutes tightly. Then raise your hips so your body forms a straight line from your shoulders to your knees. Hold for 5 seconds.
4. Lower your body back to the starting position.

2

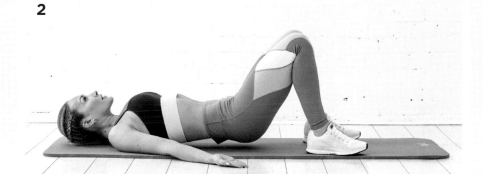

3

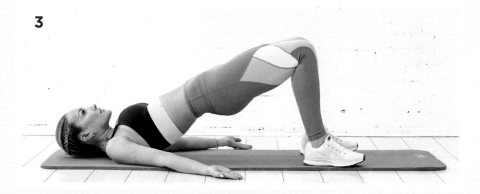

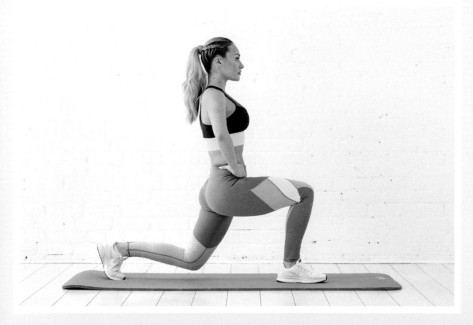

WALKING LUNGES

1. Same as Forward Lunges (see page 178) but continue the movement with your right leg forward and then your left leg forward.

FORWARD LUNGES

1. Stand tall with feet hip-width apart. Engage your core. Take a big step forward with your right leg.
2. Lower your body until your right thigh is parallel to the floor and your right shin is vertical. Press into your right heel to drive back up to the starting position.
3. Repeat on the opposite side.

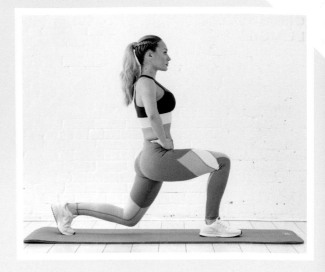

LATERAL LUNGES

1. Begin by standing with your feet shoulder-width apart.
2. Step out to the right and shift your bodyweight over your right leg, squatting to a 90-degree angle at the right knee. Keep your bum low to the floor, keeping your back as upright as possible.
3. Push off and bring your right leg back to centre to complete one rep. Repeat on your left side.

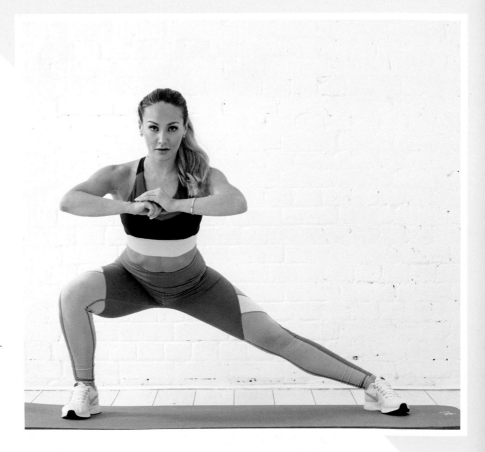

CROSS BACK LUNGES

1. Start standing with your feet shoulder-width apart.
2. Cross your right leg behind your left and lunge as far as you can to your left side. Keep your arms together in front of you to help you keep your balance.
3. Slowly return to your starting position and repeat on your left leg, lunging to your right.

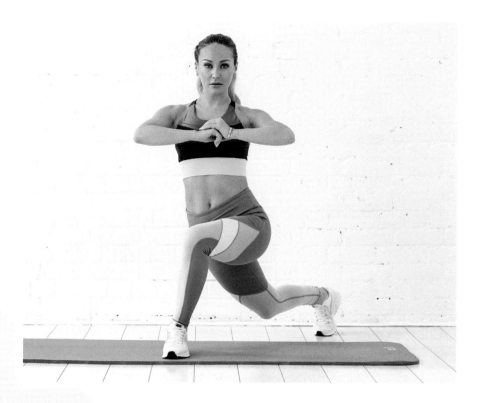

REVERSE LUNGES

1. Stand tall with your hands at your hips or overhead, engaging your core. Take a large and controlled step backward with your left foot.
2. Lower your hips so that your right thigh (front leg) becomes parallel to the floor, with your right knee positioned directly over your ankle. Your left knee should be bent at a 90-degree angle and pointing towards the floor, with your left heel lifted.
3. Return to standing by pressing your right heel into the floor and bringing your left leg forward to complete one rep.
4. Repeat on the opposite side.

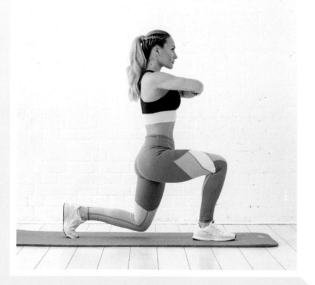

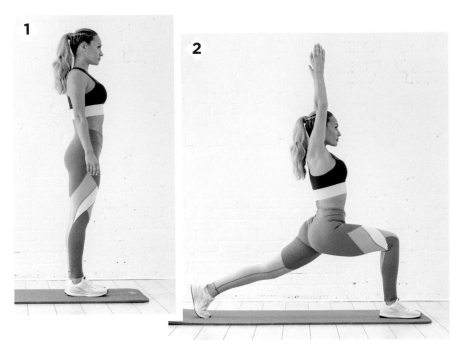

REVERSE LUNGE STRETCH

1. Follow the instructions for the Reverse Lunges on page 179 but keep your back leg extended straight out behind you.
2. Push your arms straight above your head to hold the stretch.
3. Repeat on the opposite leg.

SIDE LEG LIFTS

1. Lie on your right side and bend your right knee. Keep your left leg straight and resting on top of the right leg.
2. Push yourself up using your right arm so that your forearm is flat against the ground and your hips are raised off the floor.
3. Lift your left leg and ensure your core is engaged.
4. Repeat on the opposite side.

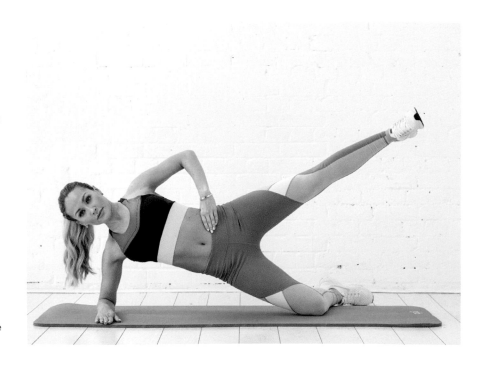

SPLIT JUMPS

1. Assume a lunge position with your right foot forward with the knee bent, and the left knee nearly touching the ground. Ensure that the front knee is over the midline of the foot.
2. Extending through both legs, jump as high as possible.
3. As you jump, bring your feet together, and switch positions so you land with your left leg forward.
4. Repeat on the opposite side.

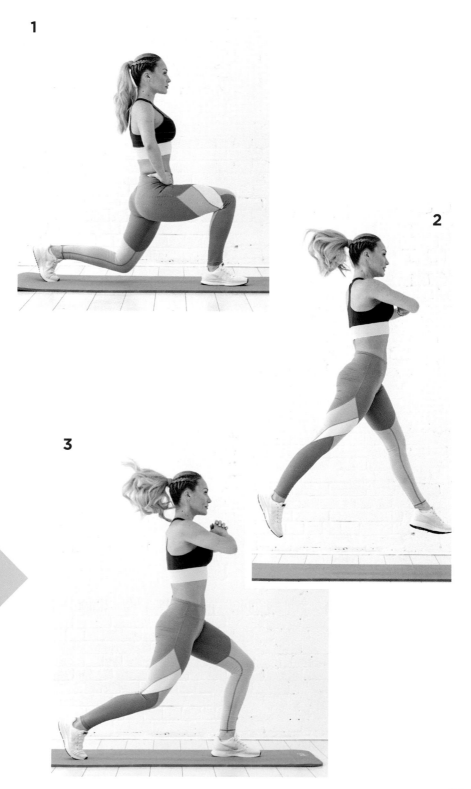

1

2

3

> 66
> Never quit, if you stumble get back up, what happened yesterday no longer matters.
> —

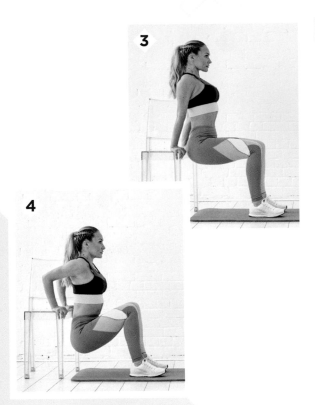

TRICEP DIPS

1. Position your hands shoulder-width apart on a secure bench or stable chair.
2. Slide your bum off the front of the bench with your legs extended out in front of you.
3. Straighten your arms, keeping a little bend in your elbows to keep tension on your triceps and off your elbow joints.
4. Slowly bend your elbows to lower your body towards the floor until your elbows are at about a 90-degree angle. Be sure to keep your back close to the bench/chair.
5. Once you reach the bottom of the movement, press down into the bench to straighten your elbows, returning to the starting position. This completes one rep.

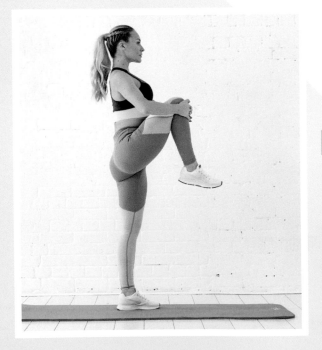

KNEE HUGS

1. Stand with your feet shoulder-width apart. Maintain a tight core throughout. Lift your right knee up and towards your chest.
2. Grab your right knee and pull it in as close as you can into your chest.
3. Slowly release the right leg to the ground. Repeat on the opposite side.

SQUAT JUMPS

1. Stand tall with your feet shoulder-width apart.
2. Start by doing a regular bodyweight squat.
3. Engage your core and jump up explosively. When you land, lower your body back into the squat position to complete one rep. Land as softly as possible, which requires control.

3

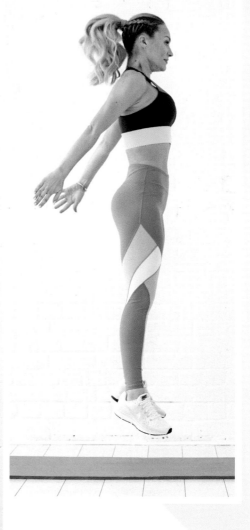

2

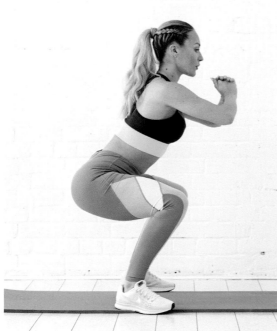

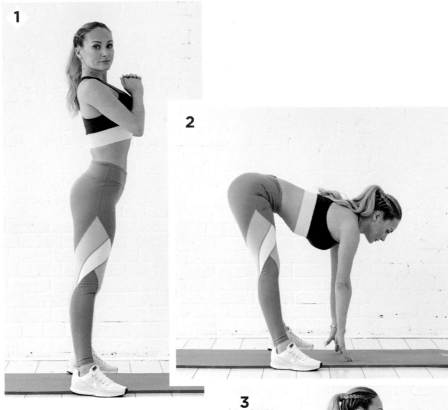

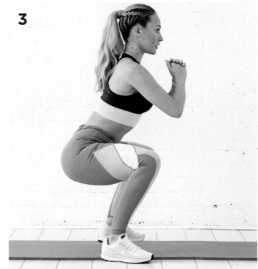

BOTTOM UP SQUATS

1. Start by standing upright with your feet shoulder-width apart and bring your hands together in front of you.
2. Hinge forward at the hips and reach down for your toes.
3. Grab your toes and drop down low into a squat.
4. In squat position reach arms high to the ceiling and return back to your starting position.

SUMO SQUATS

1. This is the same movement as for a Bodyweight Squat (see below). The difference is that you start with your legs wider apart, which emphasises the muscles on your inner thighs.

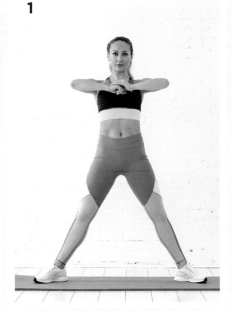

1

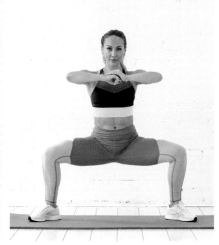

2

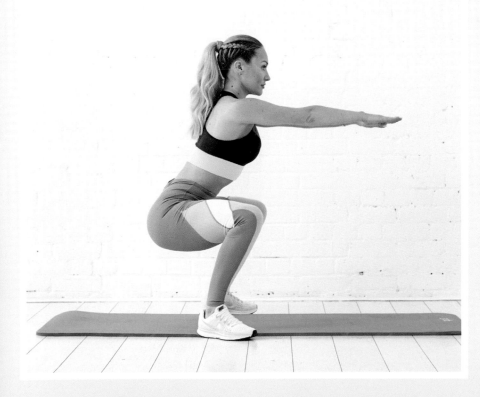

BODYWEIGHT SQUATS

1. Start with feet shoulder-width apart.
2. Extend your arms straight out in front of you with your palms facing down and keep your feet flat on the floor.
3. Slowly bend your legs and make sure your back is as straight as possible.
4. When your thighs are parallel to the floor, stand back up to finish the first rep.

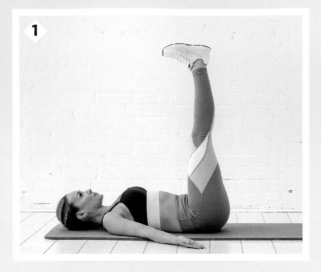

LEG RAISES

1. Start by laying flat on your back on the floor with your arms by your sides and legs stretched out next to each other. Raise your legs until they are pointing straight at the ceiling with your feet flexed.

2. Slowly lower your legs towards the floor ensuring that your core is engaged.

3. Lower them until they are just above the ground and repeat.

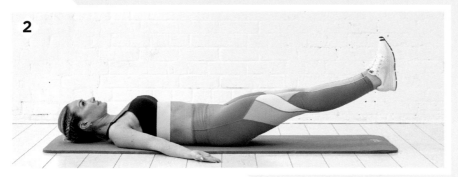

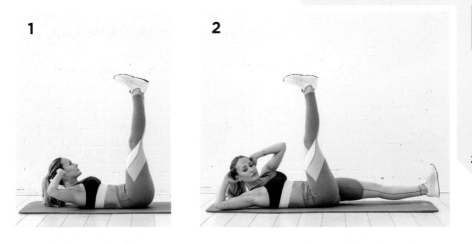

ALTERNATING LEG RAISES

1. Lie on your back on the floor and raise your legs until they are perpendicular to the floor.

2. Keeping your right leg still, lower your left leg until your heel touches the floor. Pause and then return the leg to the starting position. Repeat with the opposite leg.

2

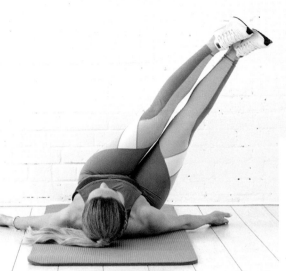

3

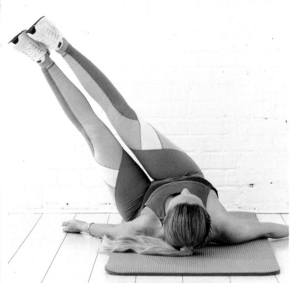

PENDULUM LEGS

1. Start by laying flat on your back, arms stretched out to the sides and your legs straight up in the air.
2. Roll your legs to one side keeping your abs tight and back straight. Hold for 2 seconds, then return to centre.
3. Roll your legs to the opposite side and back to centre to complete one rep.

SINGLE LEG HIP RAISES

1. Lie on your back with your right knee bent and right foot flat on the floor.

2. Raise your left leg up straight. Push your hips up and away from the floor, ensuring that your left leg stays elevated. Your thighs should remain at the same angle to each other.

3. Pause at the top of the movement and slowly return to the starting position. Repeat on the opposite side.

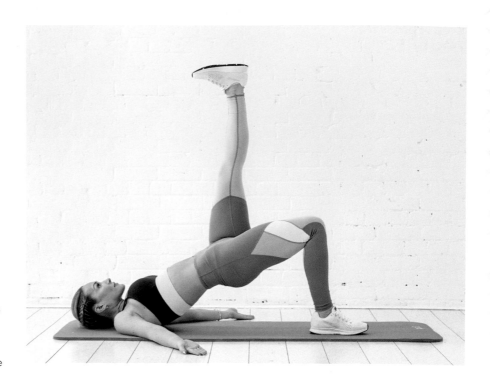

2

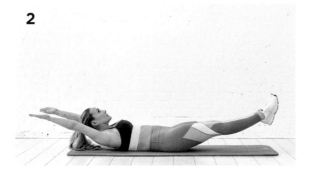

3

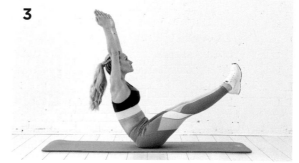

V UPS

1. Lie down on the floor and extend your arms behind your head.

2. Keep your feet together and your toes pointed towards the ceiling. Keep your legs straight and lift them up, at the same time raising your upper body off of the floor.

3. Raise your upper body further off the floor at the same time as raising your legs until you form a 'V' shape.

4. Slowly lower yourself back down to the starting position.

CRUNCH TOE TOUCHES

1. Lie on your back with your legs extended straight up at a 90 degree angle.

2. Keeping your neck straight and your eyes focused on your feet, reach up into a crunch with both hands and touch your toes. Pause and contract your core for a second, then return to your starting position.

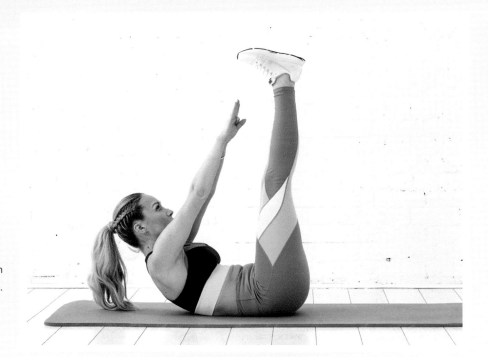

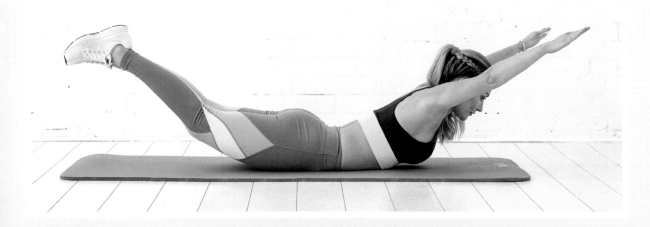

SUPERMAN

1. Lie face-down on the floor with your arms out straight in front of you. Keep your neck in a neutral position.

2. Raise your arms and gently extend the spine to raise the chest slightly off the floor to a comfortable height, and raise the legs off the ground, forming an elongated 'U' shape with your body. The arms and legs should be several inches off the floor.

3. Pause and hold this raised position for several seconds. Slowly lower back to the starting position.

FLUTTER KICKS

1. Start by lying flat on your back with your arms by your sides and your palms facing up.
2. Extend your legs fully out with a slight bend in your knees.
3. Lift your heels about 15cm off the floor. Make small, rapid up and down scissor-like motions with your legs.

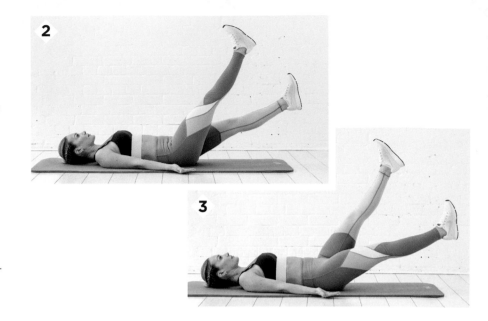

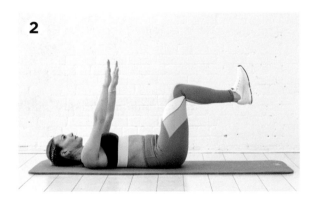

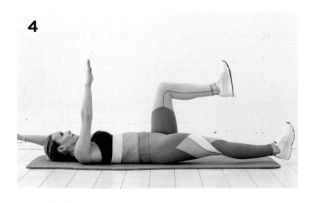

DEAD BUGS

1. Lie on your back with your arms extended in front of your shoulders.
2. Bend your hips and knees to a 90-degree angle.
3. Tighten your abs and press your lower back into the floor.
4. Slowly extend your right leg towards the floor and bring your left arm overhead. Keep your abs tight and don't let your lower back arch.
5. Slowly return your arm and leg to the starting position. Repeat with the other arm and leg.

1

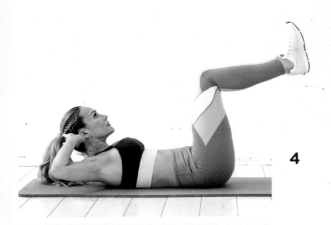

4

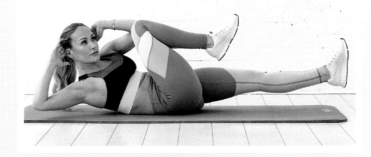

SCISSOR CRUNCHES

1. Lie on your back with your legs side by side and extended. Place your fingertips on your head just behind your ears to provide a little support for your head. Lift your head and shoulder blades off the mat. Bend your legs so that your shins are parallel to the ceiling and your feet are flexed.

2. Press your lower back firmly into the mat and slightly tuck your pelvis. Draw your belly button in towards your spine.

3. Move your legs in a vertical plane to create the scissoring action. As your right leg lifts up, your left leg lowers to hover above the mat. Keep your legs as straight as possible.

4. As your right leg rises, rotate your torso to the right, bringing your left elbow towards your right thigh. Your left shoulder blade will come higher off the ground, and your right shoulder blade may touch the mat. Return to centre as your legs pass each other, then rotate your torso to the left as your left leg rises.

gym workout guide

Get ready to burn fat, build lean muscle and challenge your body every day.

As a competitive athlete, I have spent years working on performance and fitness, testing various ways of building lean muscle and strength while burning fat. My personal fitness plan is my most effective way of achieving the best results. I found progressing from doing just cardio at the gym to lifting weights quite difficult. I am not a huge fan of lifting super-heavy weights, so I designed a fitness plan using light-to-moderate weights and sometimes just your own body weight.

In order to burn fat, you need to keep your heart rate up, so we are going to be crushing exercises back to back with little to no rest. Super sets, tri sets, plyometric training – my goal is to give you the results you want!

Remember to always challenge your body to ultimate intensity. Always welcome a challenge because it is what makes you stronger and better!

Make sure that you take a few minutes before each workout to warm up and do some dynamic stretching. Post-workout, do some Cool Down exercises (pages 213–217) and/or my full body stretching routine on pages 152–159.

legs

WARM-UP (pages 164–167)

♦ **TREADMILL WALK**
1 minute

♦ **TREADMILL SPRINTS**
5 minutes (30 seconds
intervals)

SUPER SET 1 x 3

♦ **HIP THRUSTS (see right)** x 20

♦ **RESISTANCE BAND KICK
BACKS (p. 194)** x 20

Rest 30 seconds

**BURST: RESISTANCE BAND
SQUAT JUMPS (see right)**
x 30 seconds

SUPER SET 2 x 3

♦ **KETTLEBELL SWING
(p.194)** x 20

♦ **GOBLET SQUAT (p.195)** x 20

**BURST: RESISTANCE BAND
SQUAT JUMPS (see right)**
x 30 seconds

Rest 30 seconds

SUPER SET 3 x 3

♦ **WALKING LUNGES
(p.177)** x 20

♦ **GOOD MORNINGS WITH
BAR BELL (p.195)** x 20

**BURST: RESISTANCE BAND
SQUAT JUMPS (see right)**
x 30 seconds

♦ **HIP THRUST (see right) WITH
4 SECONDS HOLD – Failure!**

1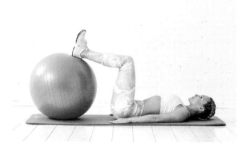

2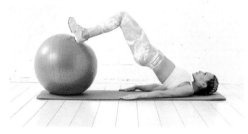

HIP THRUSTS

1. Start the move by lying on your back with your feet resting on an exercise ball. Ensure that your heels are in contact with the ball.
2. Keeping your arms flat against the ground and your shoulders pressed firmly into the floor, raise your hips whilst maintaining balance.
3. Hold when your hips are aligned with your torso and legs.

RESISTANCE BAND SQUAT JUMPS

1. Attach two bands, shoulder-width apart to a rack overhead.
2. Place your left arm through the band on your left and your right arm through the band on your right. Then take two steps back so that there is nothing above you to hit your head on. Hold each band with your hand.
3. Perform this exercise by squatting down and then exploding upwards. As you land, lower yourself into a seated squat position for a few seconds. Continue by exploding into another rep.

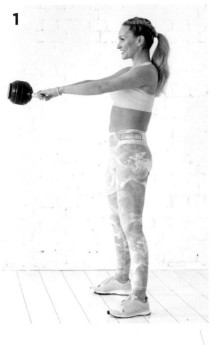

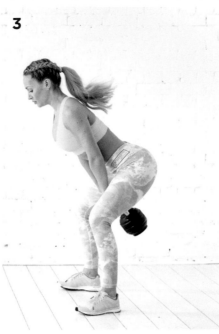

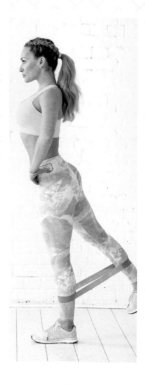

KETTLEBELL SWING

1. Start by choosing a suitable kettlebell – 8–12kg is a good starting point for women, but use a weight that you are comfortable with.
2. Stand with your feet slightly more than shoulder-width apart, toes pointed out and knees slightly bent to ensure good stability.Hold the kettlebell between your legs with both hands.
3. Bend your hips back and keep the arch in your lower back. The kettlebell should fall behind your legs – you then need to squeeze your glutes, extending through your hips and swing the weight up. Try to ensure that the movement is propelling the weight forward rather than using your arms to lift the weight.
4. From the top of the swing, allow the kettlebell to swing back between your legs, allowing your hips and knees to bend. Extend back through your hips and knees, keeping your glutes tight to reverse the momentum, and repeat. Extend your hips and knees to reverse the momentum as you immediately begin the next rep.

RESISTANCE BAND KICK BACKS

1. Start by stepping into a resistance band and position it so that it is halfway up each shin.
2. Kick back with your right foot and lock out your leg in a straight line. Release and repeat before moving onto your opposite leg.

GOBLET SQUAT

1. This is the same move as a Bodyweight Squat (page 185). Grab a dumbbell or kettlebell – choose a weight that you are comfortable with.
2. Hold the weight with both hands. Bring the weight down between your legs as you squat, ensuring that you do not bend your back to compensate for the weight.

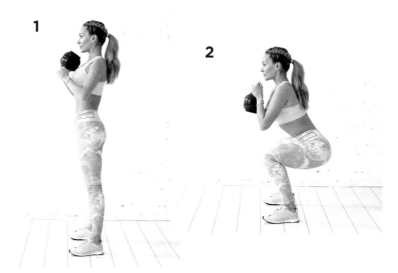

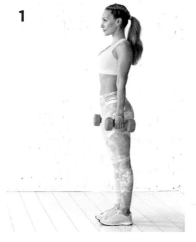

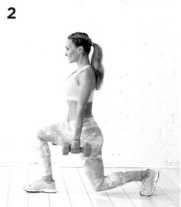

WALKING LUNGES

1. Begin standing with your feet shoulder-width apart and a dumbbell in each hand.
2. Step forward with your right leg, flexing the knees to drop your hips. Descend until your rear knee nearly touches the ground.
3. Drive through the heel of your lead foot and extend both knees to raise yourself back up.
4. Step forward with your rear foot, repeating the lunge on the opposite leg.

GOOD MORNINGS WITH BARBELL

1. Start by setting the bar on a rack that best matches your height. Once the bar is loaded, step under the bar and place the back of your shoulders across it.
2. Hold the rack bar using both arms at each side and lift it off the rack by first pushing with your legs and at the same time straightening your back.
3. Step away from the rack and position your legs using a shoulder-width (medium) stance. Keeping your legs still, move your torso forward by bending at the hips while inhaling. Lower your torso until it is parallel with the floor.
4. Begin to raise the bar as you exhale by elevating your torso back to the starting position. Repeat.

back & abs

10 MINUTES STEADY STATE CARDIO

SUPER SET 1 × 4

♦ **NARROW GRIP PULL DOWN (see right)** × 20

♦ **JUMP LUNGES (p.197)** × 20

Rest 30 seconds

SUPER SET 2 × 4

♦ **SEATED ROW (see right)** × 20

♦ **JUMP SQUATS (p.198)** × 20

Rest 30 seconds

SUPER SET 3 × 4

♦ **LAT PULL DOWN (p.197)** × 12

♦ **CABLE ROW (p.198)** × 12

Rest 30 seconds

BURST: BURPEES (p.174) × 30 seconds

SUPER SET 4 × 4

♦ **LEG RAISES (p.205)** × 25

♦ **MEDICINE BALL TOE TOUCHES (p.199)** × 25

Rest 30 seconds

TREADMILL CIRCUIT × 4

♦ **WALKING LUNGES (p.177)** × 40

♦ **SQUAT JUMPS (p.183)** × 20

♦ **SPRINT** × 30 seconds

It is never too late to start working on being the very best version of yourself.

NARROW GRIP PULL DOWN

1. Start on the pull down machine with the wide grip attachment in place. Make sure that you adjust the knee pad of the machine to fit your height.
2. Grab the bar with your hands facing forward and in a comfortable position so that you feel as though you can pull the bar down. Your hands need to be spaced out at a distance wider than the width of your shoulders.
3. As you have both arms extended in front of you bring your torso back around 30 degrees or so, keeping your chest sticking out. This is your starting position.
4. Exhale, bring the bar down until it touches your upper chest by drawing the shoulders and the upper arms down and back. Slowly release while keeping the tension and return to your starting position.

SEATED ROW

1. Start by sitting on a low pulley row machine with a V-bar. Place your feet on the front platform or crossbar provided, making sure that your knees are slightly bent and not locked. Lean over as you keep the natural alignment of your back and grab the V-bar handles.
2. With your arms extended pull back until your torso is at a 90-degree angle from your legs. Your back should be slightly arched and your chest should be sticking out. This is your starting position.
3. Keeping your torso still, pull the handles back towards your torso while keeping the arms close to it until you touch the abdominals. Exhale as you perform that movement. At that point you should be squeezing your back muscles hard.
4. Hold that contraction for a second and slowly go back to your starting position while inhaling.

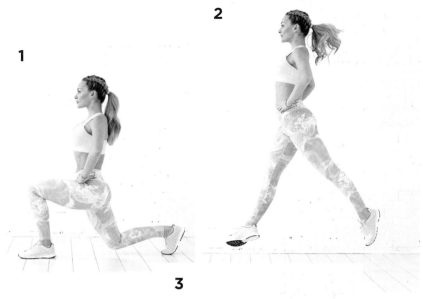

1

2

3

JUMP LUNGES

1. Start by standing tall, with your feet slightly apart. Step into a regular forward lunge, lowering your hips until both knees are bent at a 90-degree angle. Keep your upper body as straight as possible.

2. From there you have to push explosively into the air, switching the positions of your legs so that you land and can immediately drop into another lunge, but with the opposite leg forward. Try to land softly.

3. Repeat for as many reps as possible in a given time period if doing your lunges as

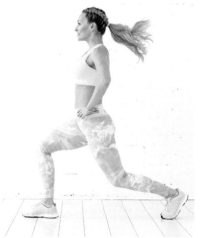

part of a circuit, or shoot for three sets of 10 on each leg. If keeping your balance and form on point during the jump lunge is tricky, make it a bit easier by holding onto a sturdy chair and shortening the length of your lunges.

LAT PULL DOWN

1. Start by sitting down on a pull-down machine with a wide bar attached to the top pulley. Make sure that you adjust the knee pad of the machine to fit your height.

2. Grab the bar with the palms facing forward and your hands slightly wider than shoulder-width apart. As you have both arms extended in front of you, bring your torso back about 30 degrees while creating a curvature on your lower back and sticking your chest out. This is your starting position.

3. As you exhale, bring the bar down until it touches your upper chest by drawing the shoulders and the upper arms down and back.

4. After a second, inhale and squeeze your shoulder blades together, slowly raising the bar back to your starting position when your arms are fully extended.

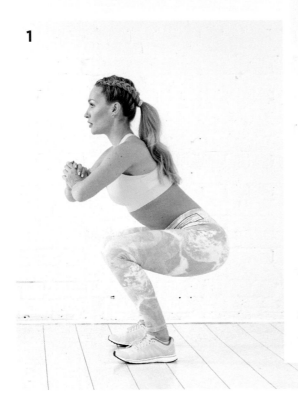

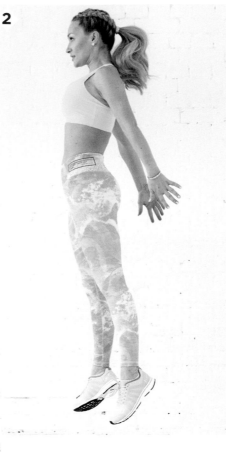

JUMP SQUATS

1. Complete the first squat as you would a normal squat (see page 185). From this position explode into the air, extending through your legs.
2. Jump explosively upwards and push your arms slightly back. Try to land softly then lower back down into the squat position.
3. Repeat.

CABLE ROW

1. Adjust the cable machine to just below chest height.
2. Start by standing in front of the cable machine with your feet shoulder-width apart and knees slightly bent. Grab a rope attachment and adjust height if needed.
3. Take a few steps back until your arms are fully extended and pull the rope back in a rowing movement keeping your chest forward and back straight.
4. Pause and slowly return to your starting position.

2

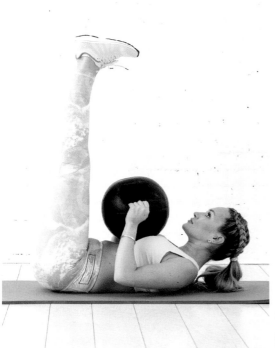

3

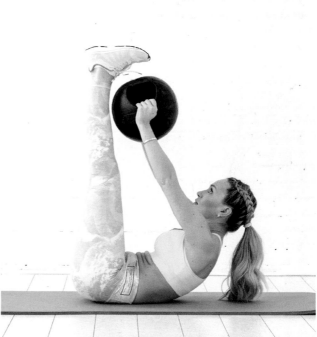

MEDICINE BALL TOE TOUCH

1. Start by lying flat on your back. Hold a medicine ball with both hands. Raise your legs up so that they are perpendicular to the ground with your feet flexed.
2. Raise the medicine ball up so that your arms are straight up above your chest. This is your starting position.
3. Begin by clenching your abs and raising your torso up so that the medicine ball nearly touches your toes.
4. Pause briefly and then slowly lower yourself back down to the starting position.

Every day you have the opportunity to wake up and become the very best version of yourself.

arms & abs

SUPER SET 1 x 3

♦ **BICEP CURL** (see right) x 20

♦ **TRICEP EXTENSION (p.201)** x 20

Rest 30 seconds

BURST: BURPEES (p.174) x 30 SECONDS

Rest 30 seconds

SUPER SET 2 x 3

♦ **DIPS ON BENCH (p.202)** x 20

♦ **TRICEP PULL DOWN (p.203)** x 20

Rest 30 seconds

SUPER SET 3 x 3

♦ **UPRIGHT ROW (p.203)** x 20

♦ **ALTERNATING FRONT RAISES (p.204)** x 20

Rest 30 seconds

BURST: SQUAT JUMPS (p.183) x 30 seconds

Rest 30 seconds

TRI SET x 3

♦ **LEG RAISES (p.205)** x 25

♦ **CRUNCHES (p.205)** x 25

♦ **PLANK SAWS (p.169)** x 20

Rest 30 seconds

BURST: MOUNTAIN CLIMBERS (p.173) x 30 seconds

Rest 30 seconds

30-SECOND SPRINTS/REST 30 SECONDS FOR 10 MINUTES

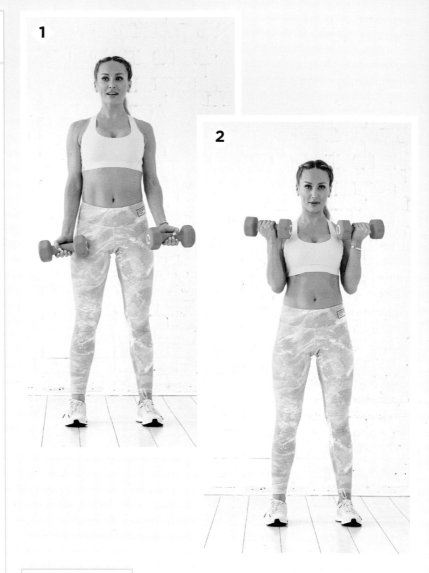

BICEP CURL

1. Start by standing up straight with a dumbbell in each hand at arm's length. Keep your elbows close to your torso and rotate the palms of your hands until they are facing forward.
2. Now, keeping the upper arms stationary, exhale and curl the weights while contracting your biceps. Continue to raise the weights until your biceps are fully contracted and the dumbbells are at shoulder level. Hold the contracted position for a brief pause as you squeeze your biceps.
3. Then, inhale and slowly begin to lower the dumbbells back to the starting position.

TRICEP EXTENSION

1. Start in a standing position with dumbbells that you feel comfortable with. Your feet should be about shoulder-width apart Slightly bend your knees and lean forward from your waist.

2. With your arms relaxed and hanging down, pull the dumbbells in towards your chest, bending from the elbow.

3. From this position, extend your arms backwards and into a straight position so that your arms are now pointing directly behind you.

4. Return to your starting position and repeat. Breathe out as you perform this step.

1

2

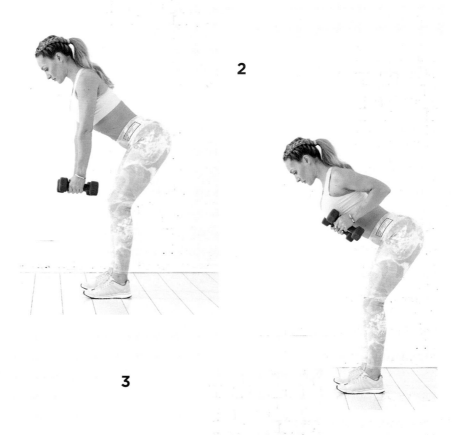

3

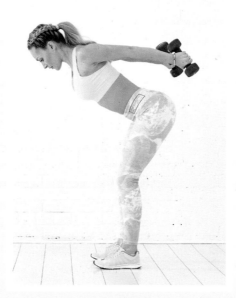

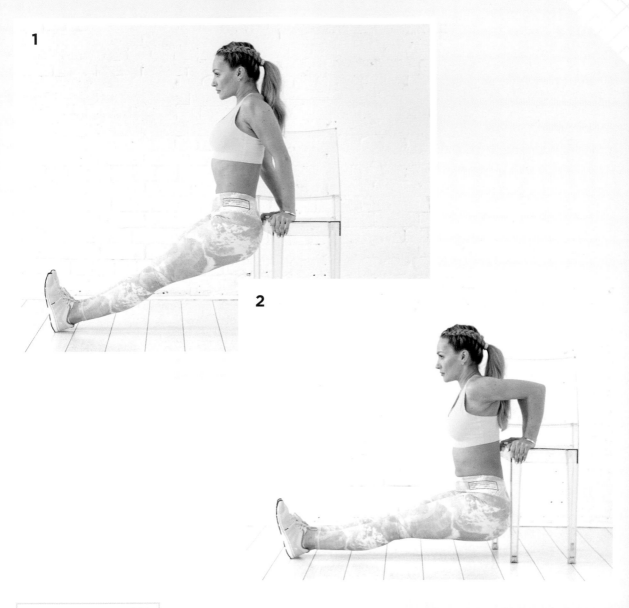

1

2

DIPS ON BENCH

1. Start with your arms slightly bent and placed firmly on a bench behind you. With the bench perpendicular to your body, and while looking away from it, hold on to the bench on its edge with the hands fully extended, separated at shoulder width. The legs will be extended forward, bent at the waist and perpendicular to your torso. This will be the starting position.

2. Slowly lower your body as you inhale by bending at the elbows until you lower yourself far enough to where there is an angle slightly smaller than 90 degrees between the upper arms and the forearms.

3. Using your triceps to bring your torso up again, lift yourself back to the starting position.

TRICEP PULL DOWN

1. Start with a straight or angled bar to a high pulley and grab it with an overhand grip at shoulder-width.
2. Standing upright with your torso straight and a very small inclination forward, bring your upper arms close to your body and perpendicular to the floor. The forearms should be pointing up towards the pulley as they hold the bar. This is your starting position.
3. Using your triceps, bring the bar down until it touches the front of your thighs and your arms are fully extended perpendicular to the floor. Your upper arms should always remain stationary next to your torso and only the forearms should move. Exhale as you perform this movement.
4. After a second, hold at the contracted position and bring the bar slowly up to the starting point. Breathe in as you perform this step.

Making yourself proud is one of the best feelings in the whole world.

UPRIGHT ROW

1. Grab a barbell or dumbbells with an overhand grip just slightly narrower than shoulder-width apart.
2. Keeping your hands as close to your body as possible pull the barbell up towards your chest.
3. Your elbows should remain pointed outwards but do not let them go above shoulder height. Hold for 1-2 seconds and then return to your starting position.

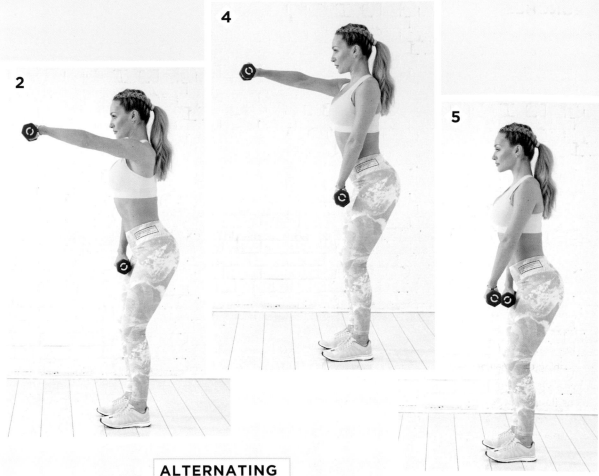

ALTERNATING FRONT RAISES

1. Start by picking up dumbbells that you are comfortable with and stand with a straight torso and the dumbbells in front of your thighs at arm's length with the palms of your hand facing your thighs. This will be the starting position.

2. Keep your torso stationary (no swinging) and lift the left dumbbell to the front with a slight bend on the elbow and the palms of your hands always facing down.

3. Continue to go up until your arm is slightly above parallel to the floor. Exhale as you complete this portion of the movement and pause for a second at the top. Inhale after the second pause.

4. Now lower the dumbbell back down slowly to the starting position as you simultaneously lift the right dumbbell.

5. Continue alternating in this fashion until you have performed the recommended amount of repetitions for each arm.

CRUNCHES

1. Start by lying flat on your back with your feet flat on the floor, or resting on a bench with your knees bent at a 90-degree angle. If you are resting your feet on a bench, place them 7.5–10cm apart and point your toes inwards so they touch.

2. Now place your hands lightly on either side of your head, keeping your elbows in. While pushing the small of your back down into the floor, begin to roll your shoulders off the floor.

3. Continue to push down as hard as you can with your lower back as you contract your abdominals and exhale. Your shoulders should come up only about 10cm off the floor. At the top of the movement, contract your abdominals hard and hold the contraction for a second.

1

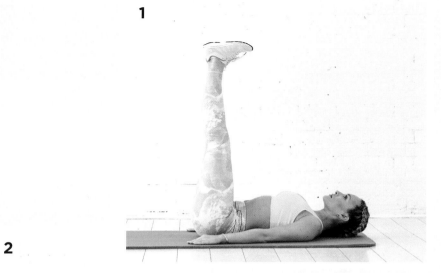

2

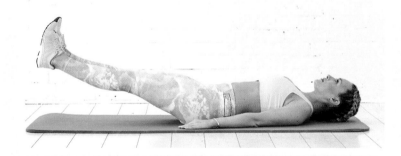

LEG RAISES

1. Start by laying flat on your back on the floor with your arms by your sides and legs stretched out next to each other. Raise your legs until they are pointing straight at the ceiling with your feet flexed.

2. Slowly lower your legs towards the floor ensuring that your core is engaged.

3. Lower them until they are just above the ground and repeat.

glutes

WARM-UP (pages 164–167)

8-MINUTE INCLINE TREADMILL WALK

SUPER SET 1 x 4

♦ **HIP THRUSTS** (p.193) x 15

♦ **BARBELL HIP THRUST** (see right) x 15

SUPER SET 2 x 4

♦ **CURTSY LUNGE** (p.208) x 20

♦ **RESISTANCE BAND SIDE-TO-SIDE STEPS** (p.207) x 20

SUPER SET 3 x 4

♦ **RESISTANCE BAND KICK BACKS** (p.194) x 20 (10 reps each leg)

♦ **SPLIT JUMPS** (p.181) x 20 (10 reps each leg)

SUPER SET 4 x 4

♦ **SUMO SQUATS** (p.185) x 20

♦ **AROUND THE WORLD BAND SQUAT JUMPS** (p.209) x 20

ROMANIAN DEAD LIFTS (p.208) **4 SETS** x 15 reps

> "
> You can never take a step back and change where you started but you can change how you will end.

BARBELL HIP THRUST

1. Start the move seated on the ground, knees raised, with the weights bench directly behind you. Have a loaded barbell over your legs, try using a pad on the bar to avoid any discomfort. The bar should be directly above your hips, lean back against the bench so that your shoulders are resting over it.
2. Drive through your feet and extend your hips vertically raising the bar. Hold at the top of your extension and slowly lower back down to your starting position.
3. Repeat.

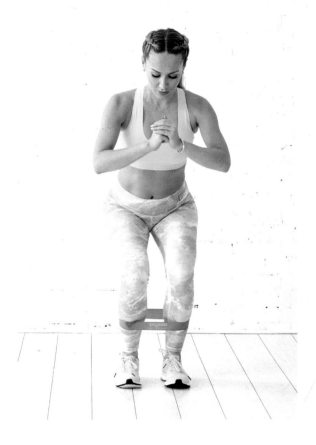

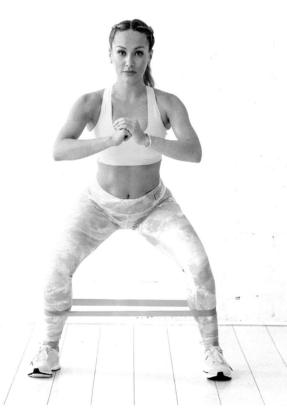

RESISTANCE BAND SIDE-TO-SIDE STEPS

1. Step inside a tied resistance band. Separate your feet so that they are hip-width apart. Place a slight bend in the knees while you keep your chest up.
2. Slowly step to the side with the right foot. Your stance should be well outside of shoulder-width.
3. Pause, then step with the left foot in the same direction as the right. Keep stepping out with the right until the set is complete, then switch sides.

CURTSY LUNGES

1. Start with your feet shoulder-width apart, holding a kettlebell at waist height in front of you with both hands. You should be looking straight forward, with your chest up and shoulders back. This will be your starting position.

2. Shift your weight to your right foot, lifting your left from the ground. While keeping your torso facing forward, place your left leg behind your right, taking a wide, lateral step behind the front leg.

3. Bend your knees, lowering your body straight down. Continue until your front knee is at approximately 90 degrees, and then drive through the heel and extend the knee and hip.

4. As you come back up, return the back leg to the starting position. Alternate the movement; switch back and forth between both sides for the stated number of repetitions.

> Fitness isn't about looking good, it's about feeling strong, flawsome and confident.

ROMANIAN DEAD LIFT

1. Start by holding a bar at hip level with palms facing down grip. Your shoulders should be back, your back arched, and your knees slightly bent. This will be the starting position.

2. Lower the bar by moving your butt back as far as you can. Keep the bar close to your body, your head looking forward and your shoulders back. Done correctly, you should reach the maximum range of your hamstring flexibility just below the knee. Any further movement will be compensation and should be avoided for this movement.

3. At the bottom of your range of motion, return to the starting position by driving the hips forward to stand up tall.

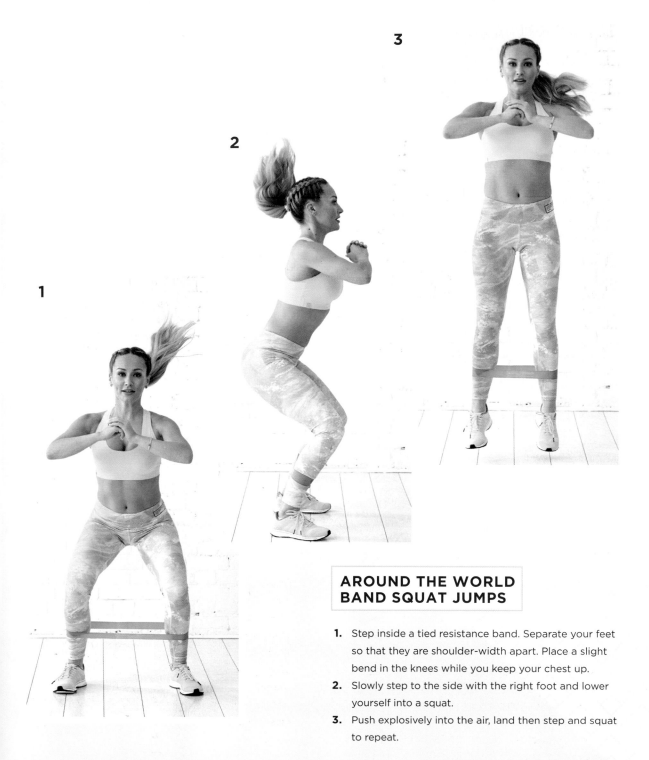

1

2

3

AROUND THE WORLD BAND SQUAT JUMPS

1. Step inside a tied resistance band. Separate your feet so that they are shoulder-width apart. Place a slight bend in the knees while you keep your chest up.
2. Slowly step to the side with the right foot and lower yourself into a squat.
3. Push explosively into the air, land then step and squat to repeat.

full body

- **JUMPING LUNGES** (see right)
  45 seconds x 4

- **HIGH KNEE MARCH** (p.165)
  45 seconds x 4

- **STEP UPS** (p.211)
  45 seconds x 4

- **LEG RAISES** (p.205)
  45 seconds x 4

- **PRESS-UPS** (p.212)
  45 seconds x 4

- **REVERSE LUNGES** (p.179)
  45 seconds x 4

- **MEDICINE BALL TOE TOUCH**
  (p.199) 45 seconds x 4

- **PLANK SAWS** (p.169)
  45 seconds x 4

- **STEADY STATE CARDIO** x
  20 minutes

JUMPING LUNGES

1. Start by standing tall, with your feet slightly apart. Step into a normal forward lunge, lowering your hips until both knees are bent at a 90-degree angle. Keep your upper body as straight as possible.

2. Push explosively into the air, switching the positions of your legs so that you land and can immediately drop into another lunge but with the opposite leg facing forward.

3. Repeat the movement on the opposite side.

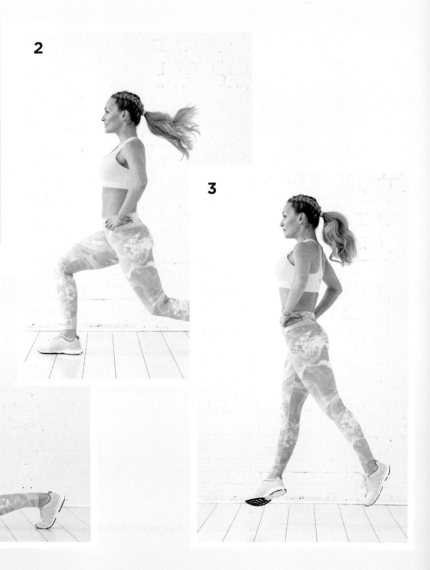

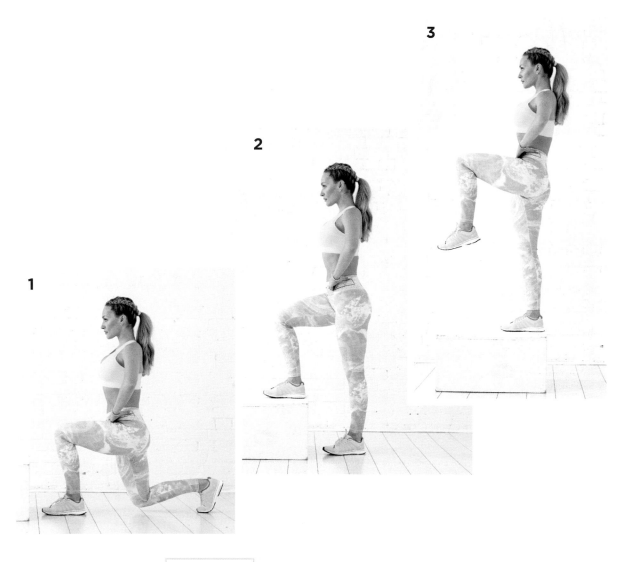

1

2

3

STEP UPS

1. Start by standing tall with your feet shoulder-width apart with an approx. 30–45cm step or block In front of you. Bring your right leg back into a reverse lunge so that your right knee nearly touches the floor. Keep your torso straight and core engaged.
2. Bring your right foot forward up onto the block.
3. Drive yourself upwards, bringing your left knee up and to the ceiling.
4. Return to start position and repeat on the opposite side.

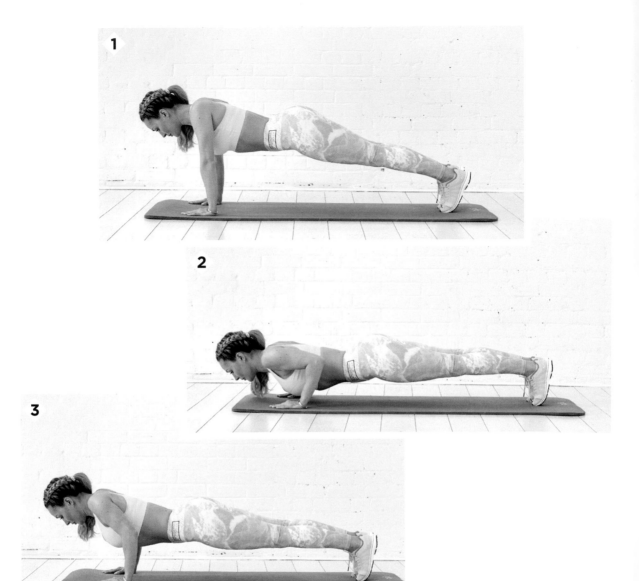

PRESS UPS

1. Start the move by lying face down on the floor face down. Bring your hands together by your shoulders and push yourself upwards until your arms are straight. Raise your hips so that your body forms a straight line and you are supporting your weight through your arms and toes.

2. Keep your elbows tucked in and bend your arms to lower yourself to the floor. Hold when you are 2.5–5cm from the floor.

3. Straighten your arms to complete the move. Repeat.

cool down

Perform each stretch for 20 secs

♦ **CHILD'S POSE** (see right)

♦ **LYING HAMSTRING STRETCH**
(p.214) LEFT/RIGHT

♦ **LYING BACK STRETCH**
(p.214) LEFT/RIGHT

♦ **DYNAMIC CHEST STRETCH**
(p.215)

♦ **KNEELING QUAD STRETCH**
(p.217)

♦ **FIGURE FOUR STRETCH**
(p.216) LEFT/RIGHT

♦ **QUAD ROCKERS** (p.217)

CHILD'S POSE

1. Start the move on your hands and knees. Push your knees wide apart whilst keeping your big toes touching. Sit up straight and rest your bum on your heels. Stretch your spine and keep it straight.

2. Exhale and allow your body to drape between your thighs. Rest your chest on the top of your thighs and allow your head to touch the floor.

3. Extend your arms with your palms facing down. Push your hands slightly into the floor so that you are pushing your bum into your heels.

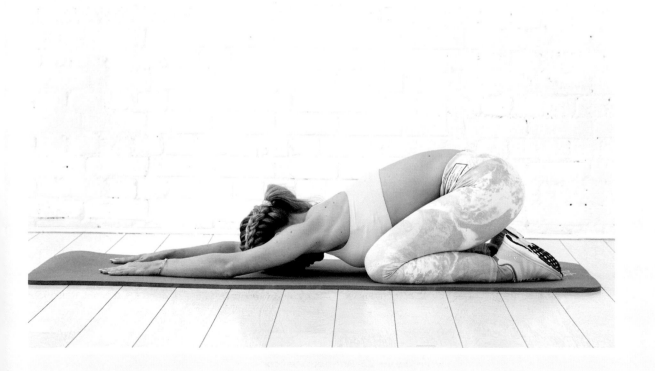

LYING HAMSTRING STRETCH

1. Start by lying on your back with your legs extended and your back straight. Keep your right leg on the floor and raise your left leg towards your chest.

2 Slowly straighten your left leg from the knee, clasp the back of your leg with both hands. Pull your leg slowly towards you while keeping both hips on the floor.

3. Hold then lower the leg to the floor and repeat on the opposite side.

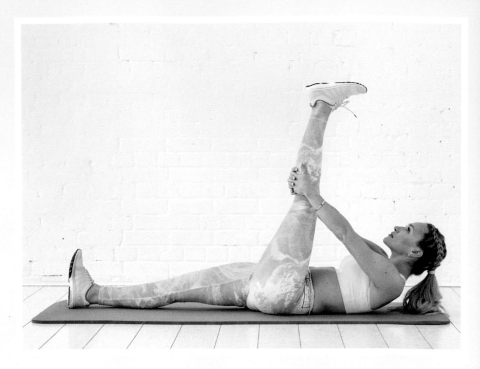

LYING BACK STRETCH

1. Start by lying on your back with legs extended flat and your back pushing into the floor.

2. Bring your right knee over your left leg so that it rests on your left side adjacent to your left hip, keeping your shoulders as flat to the floor as possible.

3. Release the left leg and repeat on the opposite side.

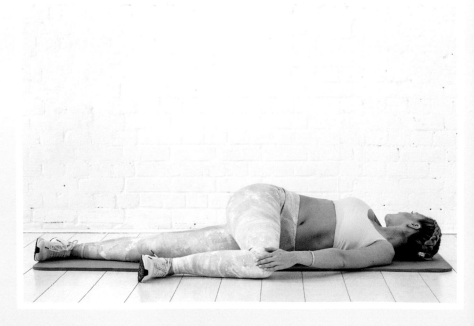

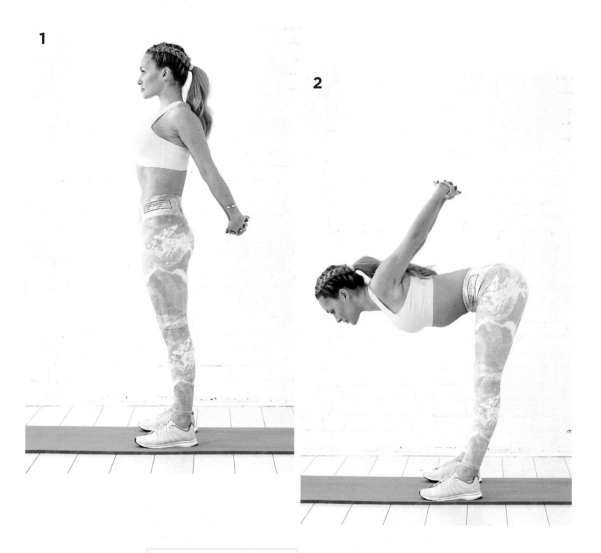

1

2

DYNAMIC CHEST STRETCH

1. Stand tall and clasp your fingers together behind your back. With your arms straight lift both arms up and away from your hips.
2. Bend from your waist to create a right angle between your legs and torso. Raise both arms up as far as you can without straining, hold for 1–2 seconds and release, continue to repeat this stretch

KNEELING QUAD STRETCH

1. Start the move by kneeling with your torso up straight.
2. Bring your right leg forward so that your right foot is flat on the ground. Stretch your left leg out behind you and ensure that your left shin keeps contact with the floor and the top of your left foot is facing down.
3. Repeat on the opposite leg and continue until you have copleted 10 stretches on each side.

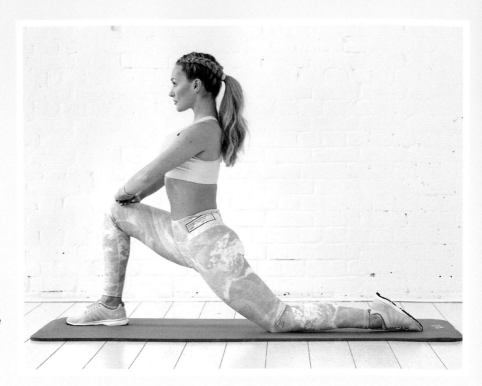

FIGURE FOUR STRETCH

1. Lie flat on your back. Bend one knee towards your torso.
2. Place your opposite ankle on the thigh of your bent leg and with both hands pull your bent leg into your chest.
3. Repeat on the opposite side.

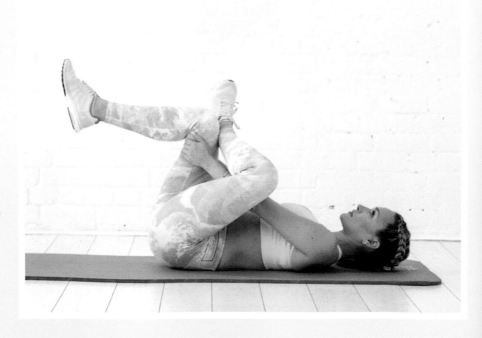

QUAD ROCKERS

1. Start the move in Child's Pose.
2. Rock your body forward pushing through your legs until you are on all fours.
3. Continue to extend forward until your body forms a straight line from your head to knees. Your wrists should be directly underneath your shoulders, arms extended, chest raised.
4. Reverse the movement rocking back into Child's Pose.

1

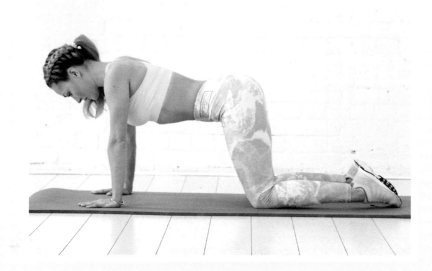

2

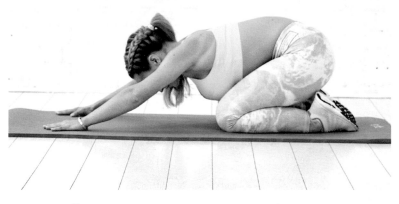

index

acknowledgements

I would like to thank each and every single person who has been part of my amazing journey and contributed to the success of my career, but I think that would call for a second book! Rather than that I would like to give a special thanks to those who have had a direct influence on my life and writing *Beat Your Bloat*.

Firstly, I would like to thank my parents Paul and Jacqueline for they have taught me everything I know and stand for. Without their love and encouragement I wouldn't be the person I am today, 'you'll get there in the end' and I guess I did. Everything I am they have helped me to be.

Thanks to Lauren Gardner for believing in me as my book agent and introducing me to Judith and Kyle from the wonderful Kyle Books. You both believed in this project from day one and I am so grateful for your support and kindness.

My book editor Vicky Orchard, who has guided me through this process and could probably write a short novel on excuses for missing deadlines.

Nikki Dupin for listening to me change my mind a million times and yet make my book so beautiful, thank you.

Tamin Jones for making my recipes look so insta perfect, I will be sharing them over and over again.

My photographer Claire Pepper for quietly capturing me as myself. Thank you.

Thank you to my golden glam squad, Maurice Flynn, Buster Knight, Nikki Wolfe and Nicholas Hardwick, we curled, we contoured and you made me feel fabulous and fearless.

My stylist Geri Doherty, for expressing me through colour and reminding us that just the colour yellow will make you smile. Oh and my bit of Irish luck.

Personal Trainer Emanuel Fritz, for keeping my energy high and form on point.

I would like to thank my management company, 84 World, for making all of this possible, you push me to create bigger goals, make me believe in myself and I love that.

Special thanks to my manager Andrew Selby, for basically having the patience of a saint. Listening to me without judgement and helping me without entitlement, you believed in me so much that this idea had no choice but to materialise.

Thank you Jenny Rose, for keeping me grounded, and for doing all that Andrew was supposed to do when I wasn't talking to him because this journey was kinda stressful.

Without the 'children' group chat, a cover may never have been chosen. I would say to my siblings, 'your greatest gift is me, but the greatest gift our parents gave us was each other'.

Joe, aka Shlomo, my younger, sometimes older brother. Four years ago you came to visit for a month... I knew having your creative mind would come in handy, now we have No Pudge Fudge and many more laughs.

Fifi, my sister, without you I wouldn't know kindness and the act of one-way sharing, although you introduced me to avocado eggs and for that I am eternally grateful.

Dan, who helped me research and now knows more about PCOS and feminine issues than any other man, don't worry you will thank me one day.

Turlough, they say the oldest children have the highest IQs but you certainly proved that to be wrong. Your grounded advice keeps us all in check, thank you for always reminding me that hard work and dedication really does pay off.

To one of my best friends who came into our lives and became part of our family, only for your great encouragement and help I wouldn't be where I am today.

And finally, most importantly, a big huge THANK YOU to all of my readers and followers. For you have been the inspiration behind writing *Beat Your Bloat*. With all the questions you asked and your own stories you have shared with me, I wanted to put everything together in one place to help you. So thank you for your encouragement and support, this one's for you!